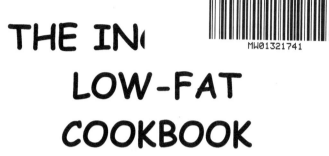

THE INCREDIBLE LOW-FAT COOKBOOK

100 super-easy recipes to prepare at home to enrich your low-fat recipe with goodness

WALLY SMITH

All rights reserved.

Disclaimer

The information contained in this eBook is meant to serve as a comprehensive collection of strategies that the author of this eBook has done research about. Summaries, strategies, tips, and tricks are only recommendations by the author, and reading this eBook will not guarantee that one's results will exactly mirror the author's results. The author of the eBook has made all reasonable efforts to provide current and accurate information for the readers of the eBook. The author and its associates will not be held liable for any unintentional error or omissions that may be found. The material in the eBook may include information by third parties. Third-party materials comprise opinions expressed by their owners. As such, the author of the eBook does not assume responsibility or liability for any third-party material or opinions. Whether because of the progression of the internet, or the unforeseen changes in company policy and editorial submission guidelines, what is stated as fact at the time of this writing may become outdated or inapplicable later.

The eBook is copyright © 2022 with all rights reserved. It is illegal to redistribute, copy, or create derivative work from this eBook whole or in part. No parts of this report may be reproduced or retransmitted in any reproduced or retransmitted in any forms whatsoever without the writing expressed and signed permission from the author.

TABLE OF CONTENTS

TABLE OF CONTENTS 3

INTRODUCTION 7

BREAKFAST 8

    1. OATMEAL BREAKFAST 9
    2. OATMEAL YOGURT BREAKFAST 11
    3. COCOA OATMEAL 13
    4. BLUEBERRY VANILLA OVERNIGHT OATS 16
    5. APPLE OATMEAL 18
    6. ALMOND BUTTER BANANA OATS 20
    7. COCONUT POMEGRANATE OATMEAL 22
    8. EGG PIZZA CRUST 24
    9. OMELET WITH VEGGIES 26
    10. EGG MUFFINS 28
    11. SMOKED SALMON SCRAMBLED EGGS 30
    12. STEAK AND EGGS 32
    13. EGG BAKE 34
    14. FRITTATA 37
    15. NAAN / PANCAKES / CREPES 39
    16. ZUCCHINI PANCAKES 41
    17. SAVORY PIE CRUST 43
    18. QUICHE 45
    19. COTTAGE CHEESE SESAME BALLS 48

APPETIZERS 50

    20. HUMMUS 51
    21. GUACAMOLE 53
    22. BABA GHANOUSH 55
    23. ESPINACASE LA CATALANA 57

24.	TAPENADE	59
25.	RED PEPPER DIP	61
26.	EGGPLANT AND YOGURT	63
27.	CAPONATA	65

SMOOTHIES 68

28.	KALE KIWI SMOOTHIE	69
29.	ZUCCHINI APPLES SMOOTHIE	71
30.	DANDELION SMOOTHIE	73
31.	FENNEL HONEYDEW SMOOTHIE	75
32.	BROCCOLI APPLE SMOOTHIE	77
33.	SALAD SMOOTHIE	79
34.	AVOCADO KALE SMOOTHIE	81
35.	WATERCRESS SMOOTHIE	83
36.	BEET GREENS SMOOTHIE	85
37.	BROCCOLI LEEKS CUCUMBER SMOOTHIE	87
38.	CACAO SPINACH SMOOTHIE	89
39.	FLAX ALMOND BUTTER SMOOTHIE	91
40.	APPLE KALE SMOOTHIE	93
41.	ICEBERG PEACH SMOOTHIE	95
42.	RAINBOW SMOOTHIE	97

DESSERTS 99

43.	CRAB CAKES	100
44.	SWEET PIE CRUST	102
45.	APPLE PIE	105
46.	FRUITS DIPPED IN CHOCOLATE	108
47.	NO-BAKE COOKIES	110
48.	RAW BROWNIES	112
49.	ICE CREAM	114
50.	APPLE SPICE COOKIES	116

SOUPS ... 118

51. CREAM OF BROCCOLI SOUP ... 119
52. LENTIL SOUP ... 121
53. COLD CUCUMBER AVOCADO SOUP ... 123
54. GAZPACHO ... 125
55. ITALIAN BEEF SOUP ... 127
56. CREAMY ROASTED MUSHROOM ... 129
57. BLACK BEAN SOUP ... 132
59. SQUASH SOUP ... 137
60. KALE WHITE BEAN PORK SOUP ... 139
61. GREEK LEMON CHICKEN SOUP ... 142
62. EGG-DROP SOUP ... 144
63. CREAMY TOMATO BASIL SOUP ... 146

MAIN DISH ... 148

64. LENTIL STEW ... 149
65. BRAISED GREEN PEAS WITH BEEF ... 151
66. WHITE CHICKEN CHILI ... 153
67. KALE PORK ... 156
68. SQUASH CAULIFLOWER CURRY ... 159
69. CROCKPOT RED CURRY LAMB ... 161
70. EASY LENTIL DHAL ... 163
71. GUMBO ... 165
72. CHICKPEA CURRY ... 168
73. RED CURRY CHICKEN ... 170
74. BRAISED GREEN BEANS WITH PORK ... 172
75. RATATOUILLE ... 175
76. BARBECUED BEEF ... 178
77. BEEF TENDERLOIN WITH SHALLOTS ... 180
78. CHILI ... 183
79. GLAZED MEATLOAF ... 186

80.	Eggplant Lasagna	188
81.	Stuffed Eggplant	191
82.	Stuffed Red Peppers with Beef	193
83.	Super Goulash	196
84.	Frijoles Charros	198
85.	Chicken Cacciatore	200
86.	Cabbage Stewed with Meat	203
87.	Beef Stew with Peas and Carrots	205
88.	Green Chicken Stew	207
89.	Irish Stew	209
90.	Hungarian Pea Stew	211
91.	Chicken Tikka Masala	213
92.	Greek Beef Stew (Stifado)	216
93.	Meat Stew with Red Beans	219
94.	Lamb and Sweet Potato Stew	222
95.	Baked Chicken Breast	225
96.	Roast Chicken with Rosemary	227
97.	Carne Asada	229
98.	Cioppino	231
99.	Flounder with Orange Coconut	234
100.	Grilled Salmon	236

CONCLUSION **238**

INTRODUCTION

A low-fat diet is one that restricts fat, and often saturated fat and cholesterol as well. Low-fat diets are intended to reduce the occurrence of conditions such as heart disease and obesity. For weight loss, they perform similarly to a low-carbohydrate diet, since macronutrient composition does not determine weight loss success. Fat provides nine calories per gram while carbohydrates and protein each provide four calories per gram. The Institute of Medicine recommends limiting fat intake to 35% of total calories to control saturated fat intake.

Although fat is an essential part of a person's diet, there are "good fats" and "bad fats." Knowing the difference can help a person make informed choices about their meals.

If you're following a healthy, balanced diet, restricting your fat intake is generally unnecessary. However, under certain circumstances, limiting the fat in your diet may be beneficial.

For example, low-fat diets are recommended if you're recovering from gallbladder surgery or have gallbladder or pancreas disease.

Low-fat diets may also prevent heartburn, cut weight and improve cholesterol.

BREAKFAST

1. Oatmeal Breakfast

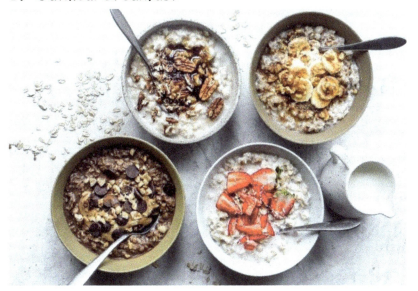

Serves 1

Ingredients

- 1 cup cooked oatmeal
- 1 teaspoons of ground flax seeds
- 1 teaspoons of sunflower seeds
- A dash of cinnamon
- Half of the teaspoons of cocoa

Directions

a) Cook oatmeal with hot water and after that mix all ingredients.

b) Sweeten if you have to with few drops of raw honey.

c) Optional: You can replace sunflower seeds with pumpkin seed or chia seed.

d) You can add a handful of blueberries or any berries instead of cocoa.

2. Oatmeal Yogurt Breakfast

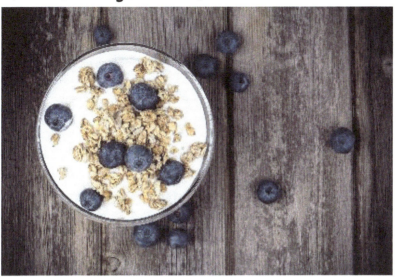

Serves 1

Ingredients

- 1/2 cup dry oatmeal
- Handful of blueberries (optional)
- 1 cup of low-fat yogurt

Directions

a) Mix all ingredients and wait 20 minutes or leave overnight in the fridge if using steel cut oats.

b) Serve

3. Cocoa Oatmeal

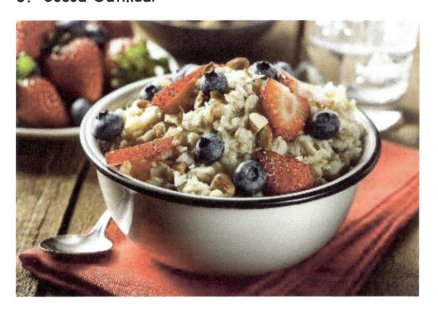

SERVES 1

Ingredients

- 1/2 cup oats
- 2 cups water
- A pinch teaspoons salt
- 1/2 teaspoons ground vanilla bean
- 2 Tablespoons cocoa powder
- 1 Tablespoons raw honey
- 2 Tablespoons ground flax seeds meal
- a dash of cinnamon
- 2 egg whites

Directions

a) In a saucepan over high heat, place the oats and salt. Cover with 3 cups water. Bring to a boil and cook for 3-5 minutes, stirring occasionally. Keep adding 1/2 cup water if necessary as the mixture thickens.

b) In a separate bowl, whisk 4 Tablespoons water into the 4 Tablespoons cocoa powder to form a smooth sauce. Add the vanilla to the pan and stir.

c) Turn the heat down to low. Add the egg whites and whisk immediately. Add the flax meal, and cinnamon. Stir to combine. Remove from heat, add raw honey and serve immediately.

d) Topping suggestions: sliced strawberries, blueberries or few almonds.

4. Blueberry Vanilla Overnight Oats

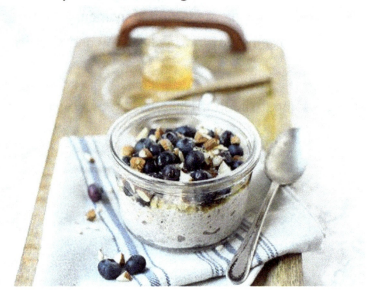

Serves 1

Ingredients

- 1/2 cup oats
- 1/3 cup water
- 1/4 cup low-fat yogurt
- 1/2 teaspoons ground vanilla bean
- 1 Tablespoons flax seeds meal
- A pinch of salt
- Blueberries, almonds, blackberries, raw honey for topping

Directions

a) Add the ingredients (except for toppings) to the bowl in the evening. Refrigerate overnight.

b) In the morning, stir up the mixture. It should be thick. Add the toppings of your choice.

5. Apple Oatmeal

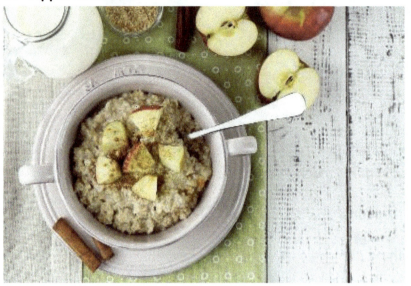

Serves 1

Ingredients

- 1 grated apple
- 1/2 cup oats
- 1 cup water
- Dash of cinnamon
- 2 teaspoons raw honey

Directions

a) Cook the oats with the water for 3-5 minutes.

b) Add grated apple and cinnamon. Stir in the raw honey.

6. Almond Butter Banana Oats

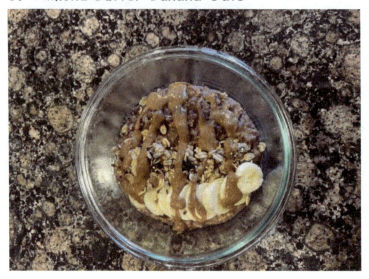

Serves 1

Ingredients

- 1/2 cup oats
- 3/4 cup water
- 1 egg white
- 1 banana
- 1 Tablespoons. flax seeds meal
- 1 teaspoons raw honey
- pinch cinnamon
- 1/2 Tablespoons. almond butter

Directions

a) Combine oats and water in a bowl. Beat the egg white, then whisk it in with the uncooked oats. Boil on stovetop. Check consistency and continue to heat as necessary until the oats are fluffy and thick. Mash banana and add to oats. Heat for 1 minute

b) Stir in flax, raw honey, and cinnamon. Top with almond butter!

7. Coconut Pomegranate Oatmeal

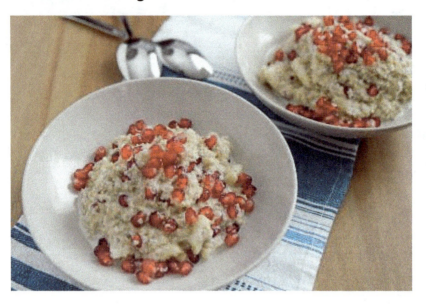

SERVES 1

Ingredients

- 1/2 cup oats
- 1/3 cup coconut milk
- 1 cup water
- 2 Tablespoons. shredded unsweetened coconut
- 1-2 Tablespoons. flax seeds meal
- 1 Tablespoons. raw honey
- 3 Tablespoons. pomegranate seeds

Directions

a) cook oats with the coconut milk, water, and salt.

b) stir in the coconut, raw honey and flaxseed meal. sprinkle with extra coconut and pomegranate seeds.

8. Egg pizza crust

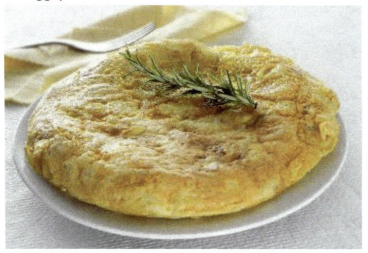

Ingredients

- 3 eggs
- 1/2 cup of coconut flour
- 1 cup of coconut milk
- 1 crushed garlic clove

Directions

a) Mix and make an omelet.
b) Serve

9. Omelet with veggies

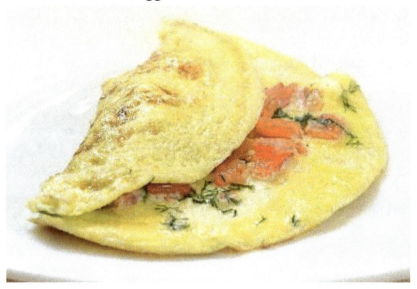

Serves 1

Ingredients

- 2 large eggs
- Salt
- Ground black pepper
- 1 teaspoons olive oil or cumin oil
- 1 cup spinach, cherry tomatoes and 1 spoon of yogurt cheese
- Crushed red pepper flakes and a pinch of dill

Directions

a) Whisk 2 large eggs in a small bowl. Season with salt and ground black pepper and set aside. Heat 1 teaspoons olive oil in a medium skillet over medium heat.

b) Add baby spinach, tomatoes, cheese and cook, tossing, until wilted (Approx. 1 minute).

c) Add eggs; cook, stirring occasionally, until just set, about 1 minute. Stir in cheese.

d) Sprinkle with crushed red pepper flakes and dill.

10. Egg Muffins

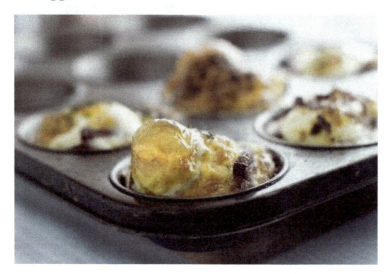

Serving: 8 muffins

Ingredients

- 8 eggs
- 1 cup diced green bell pepper
- 1 cup diced onion
- 1 cup spinach
- 1/4 teaspoons salt
- 1/8 teaspoons ground black pepper
- 2 Tablespoons water

Directions

a) Heat the oven to 350 degrees F. Oil 8 muffin cups.

b) Beat eggs together.

c) Mix in bell pepper, spinach, onion, salt, black pepper, and water. Pour the mixture into muffin cups.

d) Bake in the oven until muffins are done in the middle.

11. Smoked Salmon Scrambled Eggs

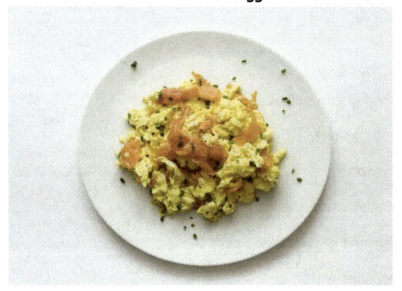

Ingredients

- 1 teaspoons coconut oil
- 4 eggs
- 1 Tablespoons water
- 4 oz. smoked salmon, sliced
- 1/2 avocado
- ground black pepper, to taste
- 4 chives, minced (or use 1 green onion, thinly sliced)

Directions

a) Heat a skillet over medium heat.

b) Add coconut oil to pan when hot.

c) Meanwhile, scramble eggs. Add eggs to the hot skillet, along with smoked salmon. Stirring continuously, cook eggs until soft and fluffy.

d) Remove from heat. Top with avocado, black pepper, and chives to serve.

12. Steak and Eggs

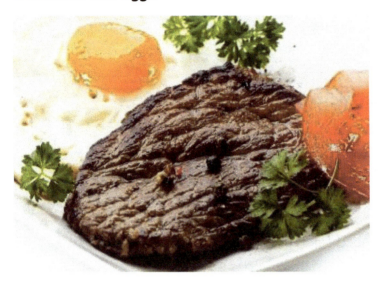

SERVES 2

Ingredients

- 1/2 lb. boneless beef steak or pork tenderloin
- 1/4 teaspoons ground black pepper
- 1/4 teaspoons sea salt (optional)
- 2 teaspoons coconut oil
- 1/4 onion, diced
- 1 red bell pepper, diced
- 1 handful spinach or arugula
- 2 eggs

Directions

a) Season sliced steak or pork tenderloin with sea salt and black pepper. Heat a sauté pan over high heat. Add 1 teaspoons coconut oil, onions, and meat when pan is hot, and sauté until steak is slightly cooked.

b) Add spinach and red bell pepper, and cook until steak is done to your liking. Meanwhile, heat a small fry pan over medium heat. Add remaining coconut oil, and fry two eggs.

c) Top each steak with a fried egg to serve.

13. Egg Bake

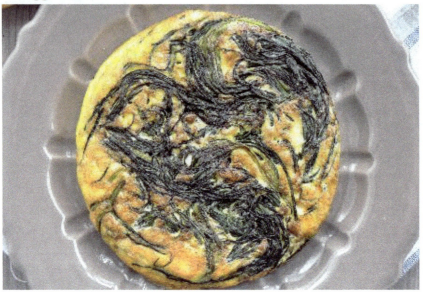

Serves 6

Ingredients

- 2 cups chopped red peppers or spinach
- 1 cup zucchini
- 2 Tablespoons coconut oil
- 1 cup sliced mushrooms
- 1/2 cup sliced green onions
- 8 eggs
- 1 cup coconut milk
- 1/2 cup almond flour
- 2 Tablespoons minced fresh parsley
- 1/2 teaspoons dried basil
- 1/2 teaspoons salt
- 1/4 teaspoons ground black pepper

Directions

a) Preheat oven to 350 degrees F. Put coconut oil in a skillet. Heat it to medium heat. Add mushrooms, onions, zucchini and red pepper (or spinach) until vegetables are tender, about 5 minutes. Drain veggies and spread them over the baking dish.

b) Beat eggs in a bowl with milk, flour, parsley, basil, salt, and pepper. Pour egg mixture into baking dish.

c) Bake in preheated oven until the center is set (approx. 35 to 40 minutes).

14. Frittata

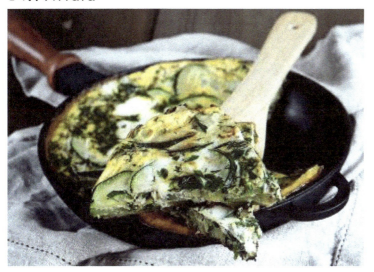

6 servings

Ingredients

- 2 Tablespoons olive oil or avocado oil
- 1 Zucchini, sliced
- 1 cup torn fresh spinach
- 2 Tablespoons sliced green onions
- 1 teaspoons crushed garlic, salt and pepper to taste
- 1/3 cup coconut milk
- 6 eggs

Directions

a) Heat olive oil in a skillet over medium heat. Add zucchini and cook until tender. Mix in spinach, green onions, and garlic. Season with salt and pepper. Continue cooking until spinach is wilted.

b) In a separate bowl, beat together eggs and coconut milk. Pour into the skillet over the vegetables. Reduce heat to low, cover, and cook until eggs are firm (5 to 7 minutes).

15. Naan / Pancakes / Crepes

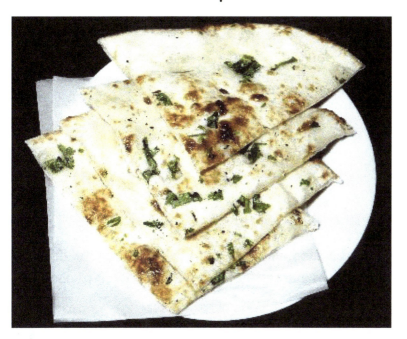

Ingredients

- 1/2 cup almond flour
- 1/2 cup Tapioca Flour
- 1 cup Coconut Milk
- Salt
- coconut oil

Directions

a) Mix all the ingredients together.

b) Heat a pan over medium heat and pour batter to desired thickness. Once the batter looks firm, flip it over to cook the other side.

c) If you want this to be a dessert crepe or pancake, then omit the salt. You can add minced garlic or ginger in the batter if you want, or some spices.

16. Zucchini Pancakes

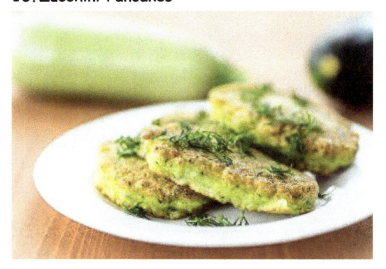

Serves 3

Ingredients

- 2 medium zucchini
- 2 Tablespoons chopped onion
- 3 beaten eggs
- 6 to 8 Tablespoons almond flour
- 1 teaspoons salt
- 1/2 teaspoons ground black pepper
- coconut oil

Directions

a) Heat the oven to 300 degrees F.

b) Grate the zucchini into a bowl and stir in the onion and eggs. Stir in 6 Tablespoons of the flour, salt, and pepper.

c) Heat a large sauté pan over medium heat and add coconut oil in the pan. When the oil is hot, lower the heat to medium-low and add batter into the pan. Cook the pancakes about 2 minutes on each side, until browned. Place the pancakes in the oven.

17. Savory Pie Crust

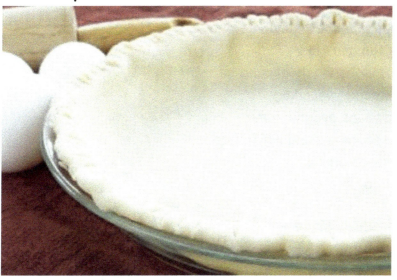

Ingredients

- 11/4 cups blanched almond flour
- 1/3 cup tapioca flour
- 3/4 teaspoons finely ground sea salt
- 3/4 teaspoons paprika
- 1/2 teaspoons ground cumin
- 1/8 teaspoons ground white pepper
- 1/4 cup coconut oil
- 1 large egg

Directions

a) Place almond flour, tapioca flour, sea salt, vanilla, egg and coconut sugar (if you use coconut sugar) in the bowl of a food processor. Process 2-3 times to combine. Add oil and raw honey (if you use raw honey) and pulse with several one-second pulses and then let the food processor run until the mixture comes together. Move dough onto a plastic wrap sheet. Wrap and then press the dough into a 9-inch disk. Refrigerate for 30 minutes.

b) Remove plastic wrap. Press dough onto the bottom and up the sides of a 9-inch buttered pie dish. Crimp a little bit the edges of crust. Cool in the refrigerator for 20 minutes. Put the oven rack to middle position and preheat oven to 375F. Put in the oven and bake until golden brown.

18. Quiche

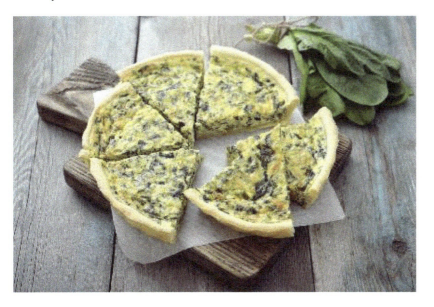

SERVES 2-3

Ingredients

- 1 Precooked and cooled Savory Pie Crust
- 8 ounces organic spinach, cooked and drained
- 6 ounces cubed pork
- 2 medium shallots, thinly sliced and sautéed
- 4 large eggs
- 1 cup coconut milk
- 3/4 teaspoons salt
- 1/4 teaspoons freshly ground black pepper

Directions

a) Brown the pork in coconut oil and then add the spinach and shallots. Set aside once done.

b) Preheat oven to 350F. In a large bowl, combine eggs, milk, salt and pepper. Whisk until foamy. Add in about 3/4 of the drained filling mixture, reserving the other 1/4 to "top" the quiche. Pour egg mixture into crust and place remaining filling on top of the quiche.

c) Place quiche in oven in the center of the middle rack and bake undisturbed for 45 to 50 minutes.

19. Cottage Cheese Sesame Balls

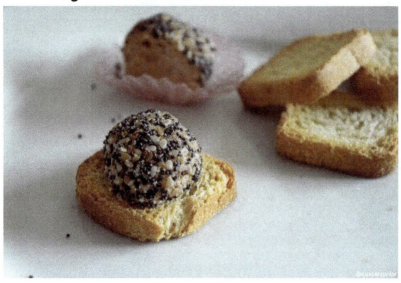

Ingredients

- 16 ounce farmers cheese or cottage cheese
- 1 cup finely chopped almonds
- 1 and 1/2 cups oatmeal

Directions

a) In a large bowl, combine blended cottage cheese, almonds and oatmeal.
b) Make balls and roll in sesame seeds mix.

APPETIZERS

20. Hummus

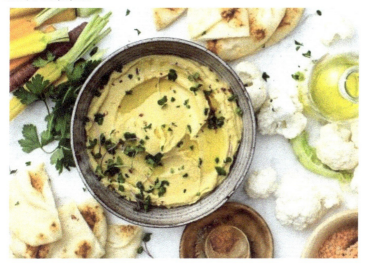

Ingredients

- 2 cups cooked chickpeas (garbanzo beans)
- 1/4 cup (59 ml) fresh lemon juice
- 1/4 cup (59 ml) tahini
- Half of a large garlic clove, minced
- 2 Tablespoons olive oil or cumin oil, plus more for serving
- 1/2 to 1 teaspoons salt
- 1/2 teaspoons ground cumin
- 2 to 3 Tablespoons water
- Dash of ground paprika for serving

Directions

a) Combine tahini and lemon juice and blend for 1 minute. Add the olive oil, minced garlic, cumin and the salt to tahini and lemon mixture. Process for 30 seconds, scrape sides and then process 30 seconds more.

b) Add half of the chickpeas to the food processor and process for 1 minute. Scrape sides, add remaining chickpeas and process for 1 to 2 minutes.

c) Transfer the hummus into a bowl then drizzle about 1 Tablespoons of olive oil over the top and sprinkle with paprika.

21. Guacamole

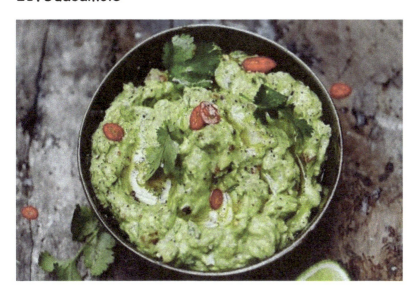

Ingredients

- 4 ripe avocados
- 3 Tablespoons freshly squeezed lemon juice (1 lemon)
- 8 dashes hot pepper sauce
- 1/2 cup diced onion
- 1 large garlic clove, minced
- 1 teaspoons salt
- 1 teaspoons ground black pepper
- 1 medium tomato, seeded, and small-diced

Directions

a) Cut the avocados in half, remove the pits, and scoop the flesh out.

b) Immediately add the lemon juice, hot pepper sauce, garlic, onion, salt, and pepper and toss well. Dice avocados. Add the tomatoes.

c) Mix well and taste for salt and pepper.

22. Baba Ghanoush

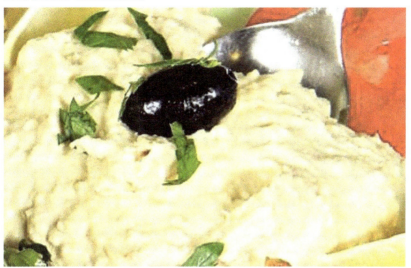

Ingredients

- 1 large eggplant
- 1/4 cup tahini, plus more as needed
- 3 garlic cloves, minced
- 1/4 cup fresh lemon juice, plus more as needed
- 1 pinch ground cumin
- salt, to taste
- 1 Tablespoons extra-virgin olive oil or avocado oil
- 1 Tablespoons chopped flat-leaf parsley
- 1/4 cup brine-cured black olives, such as Kalamata

Directions

a) Grill eggplant for 10 to 15 minutes. Heat the oven (375 F).

b) Put the eggplant to a baking sheet and bake 15-20 minutes or until very soft. Remove from the oven, let cool, and peel off and discard the skin. Put the eggplant flesh in a bowl. Using a fork, mash the eggplant to a paste.

c) Add the 1/4 cup tahini, garlic, cumin, 1/4 cup lemon juice and mix well. Season with salt to taste. Transfer the mixture to a serving bowl and spread with the back of a spoon to form a shallow well. Drizzle the olive oil over the top and sprinkle with the parsley.

23. Espinacase la Catalana

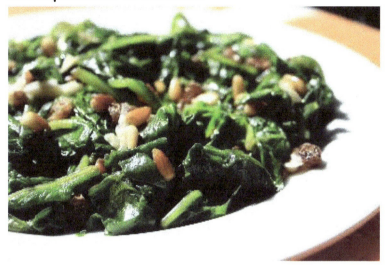

Serves 4

Ingredients

- 2 cups spinach
- 2 cloves garlic
- 3 Tablespoons cashews
- 3 Tablespoons dried currants
- olive oil or avocado oil

Directions

a) Wash the spinach and trim off the stems. Steam the spinach for few minutes.

b) Peel and slice the garlic. Pour a few tablespoons of olive oil and cover the bottom of a frying pan. Heat pan on medium and sauté garlic for 1-2 minutes.

c) Add the cashews and the currants to the pan and continue to sauté for 1 minute. Add the spinach and mix well, coating with oil. Salt to taste.

24. Tapenade

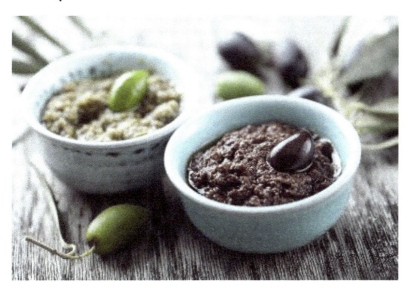

Ingredients

- 1/2 pound pitted mixed olives
- 2 anchovy fillets, rinsed
- 1 small clove garlic, minced
- 2 Tablespoons capers
- 2 to 3 fresh basil leaves
- 1 Tablespoons freshly squeezed lemon juice
- 2 Tablespoons extra-virgin olive oil or cumin oil

Directions

a) Rinse the olives in cool water.
b) Place all ingredients in the bowl of a food processor. Process to combine, until it becomes a coarse paste.
c) Transfer to a bowl and serve

25. Red Pepper Dip

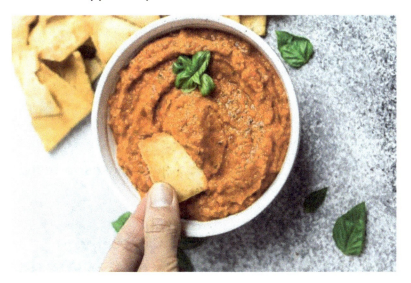

Ingredients

- 1 pound red peppers
- 1 cup farmers' cheese
- 1/4 cup virgin olive oil or avocado oil
- 1 Tablespoons minced garlic
- Lemon juice, salt, basil, oregano, red pepper flakes to taste.

Directions

a) Roast the peppers. Cover them and cool for about 15 minutes. Peel the peppers and remove the seeds and stems.
b) Chop the peppers.
   Transfer the peppers and garlic to a food processor and process until smooth.
c) Add the farmers' cheese and garlic and process until smooth.
d) With the machine running, add olive oil and lemon juice. Add the basil, oregano, red pepper flakes, and 1/4 teaspoons salt, and process until smooth.
e) Adjust the seasoning, to taste. Pour to a bowl and refrigerate.

26. Eggplant and Yogurt

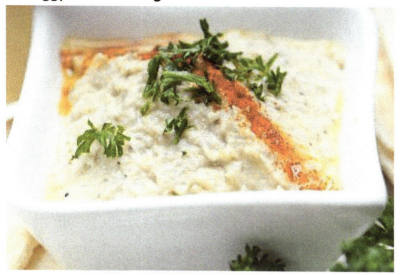

Ingredients

- 1 pound chopped eggplant
- 3 unpeeled shallots
- 3 unpeeled garlic cloves

Directions

a) Mix 1 pound chopped eggplant, 3 unpeeled shallots and 3 unpeeled garlic cloves with 1/4 cup olive oil, salt and pepper on a baking sheet.

b) Roast at 400 degrees for half an hour. Cool and squeeze the shallots and garlic from their skins and chop. Mix with the eggplant, almond, 1/2 cup plain yogurt, dill and salt and pepper.

27. Caponata

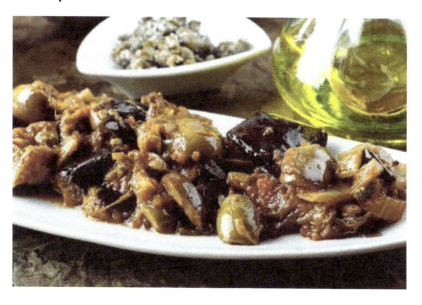

SERVES 3-4

Ingredients

- coconut oil
- 2 large eggplants, cut into large chunks
- 1 teaspoons dried oregano
- Sea salt
- Freshly ground black pepper
- 1 small onion, peeled and finely chopped
- 2 cloves garlic, peeled and finely sliced
- 1 small bunch fresh flat-leaf parsley, leaves picked and stalks finely chopped
- 2 Tablespoons salted capers, rinsed, soaked and drained
- 1 handful green olives, stones removed
- 2-3 Tablespoons lemon juice
- 5 large ripe tomatoes, roughly chopped
- coconut oil
- 2 Tablespoons slivered almonds, lightly toasted, optional

Directions

a) Heat coconut oil in a pan and add eggplant, oregano and salt. Cook on a high heat for around 4 or 5 minutes. Add the onion, garlic and parsley stalks and continue cooking for another few minutes. Add drained capers and the olives and lemon juice. When all the juice has evaporated, add the tomatoes and simmer until tender.

b) Season with salt and olive oil to taste before serving. Sprinkle with almonds.

SMOOTHIES

28. Kale Kiwi Smoothie

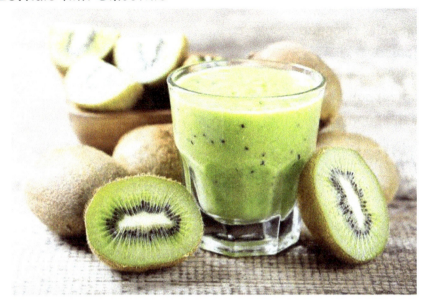

Ingredients

- 1 cup Kale, chopped
- 2 Apples
- 3 Kiwis
- 1 tablespoon flax seeds
- 1 tablespoon royal jelly
- 1 cup crushed ice

Directions

a) Combine in blender
b) Serve

29. Zucchini Apples Smoothie

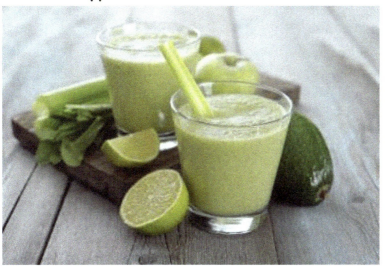

Ingredients

- 1/2 cup zucchini
- 2 Apples
- 3/4 avocado
- 1 stalk Celery
- 1 Lemon
- 1 Tablespoons Spirulina
- 1 1/2 cups crushed ice

Directions

a) Combine in blender

b) Serve

30. Dandelion Smoothie

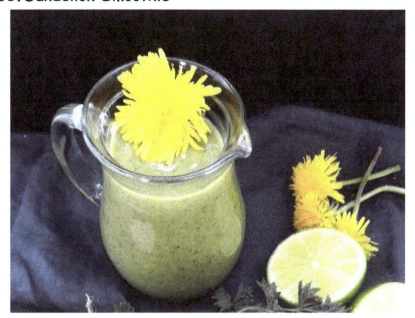

Ingredients

- 1 cup Dandelion greens
- 1 cup Spinach
- ½ cup tahini
- 1 Red Radish
- 1 Tablespoons chia seeds
- 1 cup lavender tea

Directions

a) Combine in blender
b) Serve

31. Fennel Honeydew Smoothie

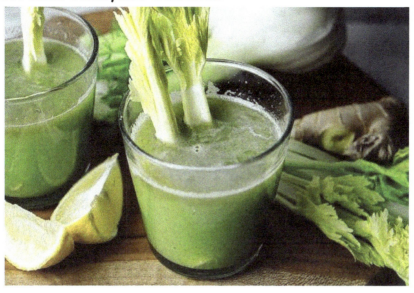

Ingredients

- ½ cup fennel
- 1 cup Broccoli
- 1 Tablespoons Cilantro
- 1 cup Honeydew
- 1 cup crushed ice
- 1 Tablespoons Chlorella

Directions

a) Combine in blender
b) Serve

32. Broccoli Apple Smoothie

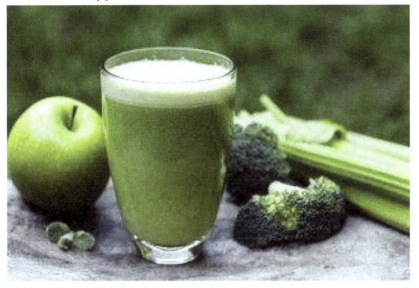

Ingredients

- 1 Apple
- 1 cup Broccoli
- 1 Tablespoons Cilantro
- 1 Celery stalk
- 1 cup crushed ice
- 1 Tablespoons crushed Seaweed

Directions

a) Combine in blender
b) Serve

33. Salad Smoothie

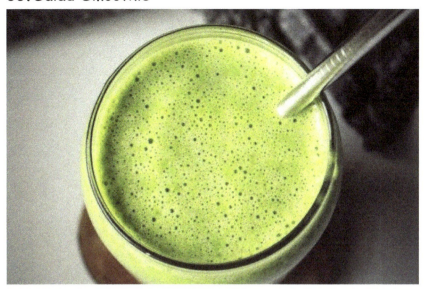

Ingredients

- 1 cup spinach
- ½ cucumber
- 1/2 small onion
- 2 tablespoons Parsley
- 2 tablespoons lemon juice
- 1 cup crushed ice
- 1 Tablespoons olive oil or cumin oil
- ¼ cup Wheatgrass

Directions

a) Combine in blender

b) Serve

34. Avocado Kale Smoothie

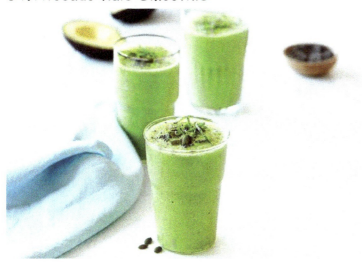

Ingredients

- 1 cup Kale
- ½ Avocado
- 1 cup Cucumber
- 1 Celery Stalk
- 1 Tablespoons chia seeds
- 1 cup chamomile tea
- 1 Tablespoons Spirulina

Directions

a) Combine in blender
b) Serve

35. Watercress Smoothie

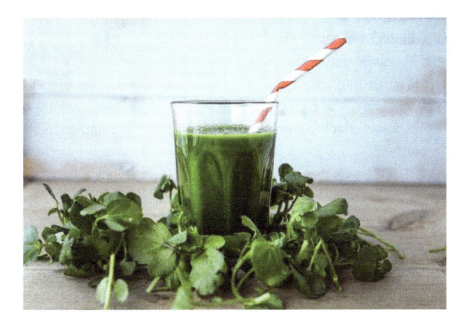

Ingredients

- 1 cup Watercress
- ½ cup almond butter
- 2 small cucumbers
- 1 cup coconut milk
- 1 Tablespoons Chlorella
- 1 Tablespoons Black cumin seeds – sprinkle on top and garnish with parsley

Directions

a) Combine in blender

b) Serve

36. Beet Greens Smoothie

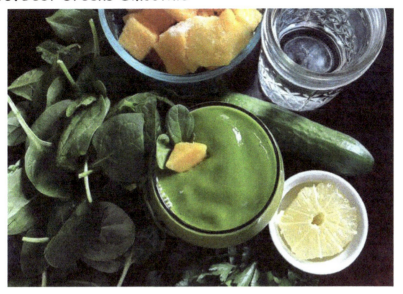

Ingredients

- 1 cup Beet Greens
- 2 Tablespoons Pumpkin seeds butter
- 1 cup Strawberry
- 1 Tablespoons Sesame seeds
- 1 Tablespoons hemp seeds
- 1 cup chamomile tea

Directions

a) Combine in blender
b) Serve

37. Broccoli Leeks Cucumber smoothie

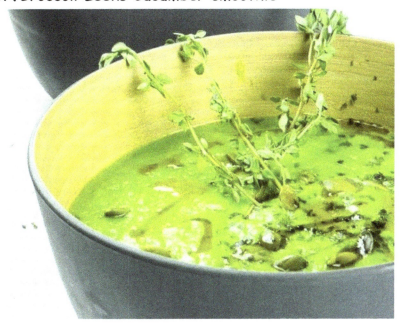

Ingredients

- 1 cup Broccoli
- 2 Tablespoons Cashew butter
- 2 Leeks
- 2 Cucumbers
- 1 Lime
- ½ cup Lettuce
- ½ cup Leaf Lettuce
- 1 Tablespoons Matcha
- 1 cup crushed ice

Directions

a) Combine in blender
b) Serve

38. Cacao Spinach Smoothie

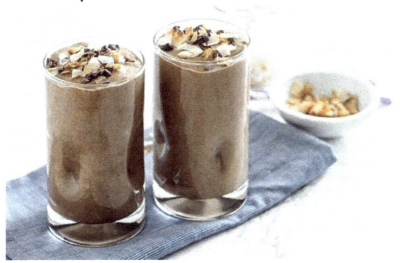

Ingredients

- 2 cups spinach
- 1 cup blueberries, frozen
- 1 tablespoon dark cocoa powder
- ½ cup unsweetened almond milk
- 1/2 cup crushed ice
- 1 teaspoon raw honey
- 1 Tablespoons Matcha powder

Directions

a) Combine in blender

b) Serve

39. Flax Almond Butter Smoothie

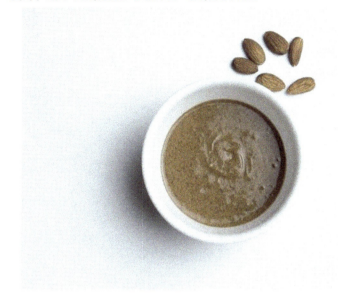

Ingredients

- ½ cup plain yogurt
- 2 tablespoons almond butter
- 2 cups spinach
- 1 banana, frozen
- 3 strawberries
- 1/2 cup crushed ice
- 1 teaspoon flax seeds

Directions

a) Combine in blender
b) Serve

40. Apple Kale Smoothie

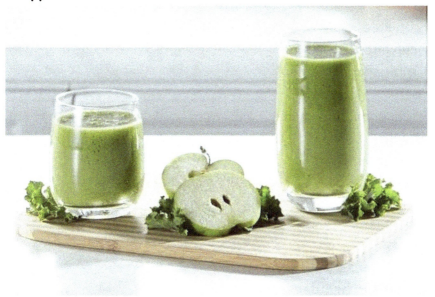

Ingredients

- 1 cup kale
- ½ cup coconut milk
- 1 Tablespoons Maca
- 1 banana, frozen
- ¼ teaspoon cinnamon
- 1 Apple
- Pinch of nutmeg
- 1 clove
- 3 ice cubes

Directions

a) Combine in blender
b) Serve

41. Iceberg Peach Smoothie

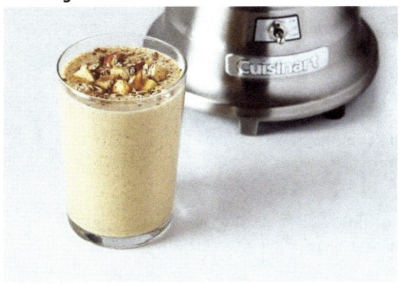

Ingredients

- 1 cup Iceberg lettuce
- 1 Banana
- 1 peach
- 1 Brazil Nut
- 1 Mango
- 1 cup Kombucha
- Top with hemp seeds

Directions

a) Combine in blender
b) Serve

42. Rainbow Smoothie

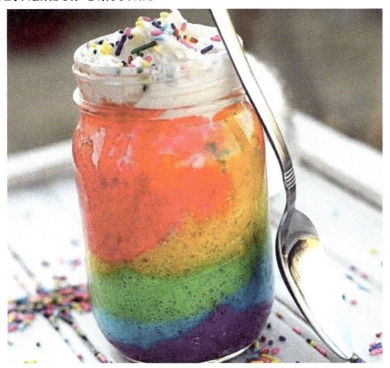

Directions

a) Blend 1 Large beet with some crushed ice
b) Blend 3 carrots with some crashed ice
c) Blend 1 cucumber, 1 cup of leaf lettuce and $\frac{1}{2}$ cup Wheatgrass
d) Serve them separate to preserve the distinct color
e) Serve

DESSERTS

43. Crab Cakes

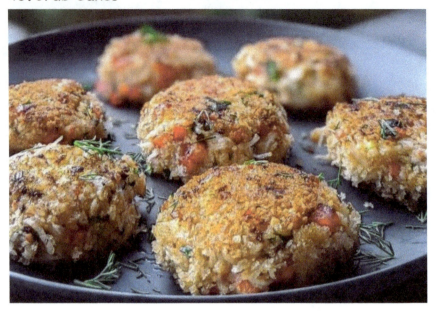

Serves 6-8

Ingredients

- 3 lbs. crabmeat
- 3 beaten eggs
- 3 cups flax seeds meal
- 3 Tablespoons mustard
- 2 Tablespoons grated horseradish
- 1/2 cup coconut oil
- 1 teaspoon. lemon rind
- 3 Tablespoons lemon juice
- 2 Tablespoons parsley
- 1/2 teaspoons cayenne pepper
- 2 teaspoons fish sauce

Directions

a) In medium bowl combine all ingredients except oil.
b) Shape in to smallish hamburgers. In fry pan heat oil and cook patties for 3-4 minutes on each side or until golden brown.
c) Optionally, bake them in the oven.
d) Serve as appetizers or as main course with large fiber salad.

44. Sweet pie crust

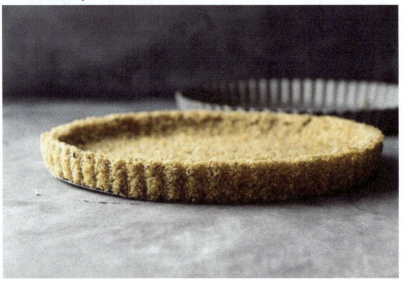

Ingredients

- 1 1/3 cups blanched almond flour
- 1/3 cup tapioca flour
- 1/2 teaspoons sea salt
- 1 large egg
- 1/4 cup coconut oil
- 2 Tablespoons coconut sugar or raw honey
- 1 teaspoons of ground vanilla bean

Directions

a) Place almond flour, tapioca flour, sea salt, vanilla, egg and coconut sugar (if you use coconut sugar) in the bowl of a food processor. Process 2-3 times to combine. Add oil and raw honey (if you use raw honey) and pulse with several one-second pulses and then let the food processor run until the mixture comes together. Pour dough onto a sheet of plastic wrap. Wrap and then press the dough into a 9-inch disk. Refrigerate for 30 minutes.

b) Remove plastic wrap. Press dough onto the bottom and up the sides of a 9-inch buttered pie dish. Crimp a little bit the edges of crust. Cool in the refrigerator for 20 minutes.

Put the oven rack to middle position and preheat oven to 375F. Put in the oven and bake until golden brown.

45. Apple Pie

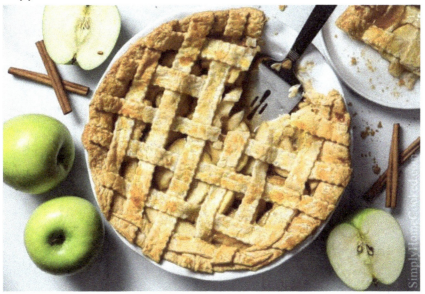

Serving Size: Serves 8

Ingredients

- 2 Tablespoons coconut oil
- 9 sour apples, peeled, cored and cut into 1/4-inch thick slices
- 1/4 cup coconut sugar or raw honey
- 1/2 teaspoons cinnamon
- 1/8 teaspoons sea salt
- 1/2 cup coconut milk
- 1 cup ground nuts and seeds

Directions

a) Filling: Melt coconut oil in a large pot over medium heat. Add apples, coconut sugar or raw honey, cinnamon and sea salt.

b) Increase heat to medium-high and cook, stirring occasionally, until apples release their moisture and sugar is melted. Pour coconut milk or cream over apples and continue to cook until apples are soft and liquid has thickened, about 5 minutes, stirring occasionally.

c) Pour the filling into the crust and then top with topping. Place a pie shield over the edges of the crust to avoid burning. Bake until topping is just turning golden brown. Cool and serve.

46. Fruits dipped in chocolate

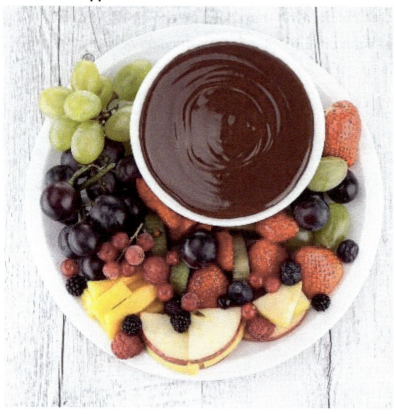

Ingredients

- 2 apples or 2 bananas or a bowl of strawberries or any fruit that can be dipped in melted chocolate

- 1/2 cup of melted chocolate \2 Tablespoons chopped nuts (almond, walnut, Brazil nuts) or seeds (hemp, chia, sesame, flax seeds meal)

Directions

a) Cut apple in wedges or cut banana in quarters. Melt the chocolate and chop the nuts. Dip fruit in chocolate, sprinkle with nuts or seeds and lay on tray.

b) Transfer the tray to the fridge so the chocolate can harden; serve.

c) If you don't want chocolate, cover fruits with almond or sunflower butter and sprinkle with chia or hemp seeds and cut it into chunks and serve.

47. No-Bake Cookies

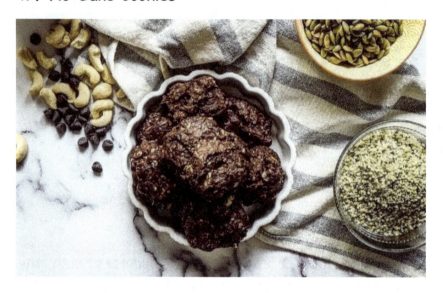

Ingredients

- 1/2 cup coconut milk
- 1/2 cup cocoa powder
- 1/2 cup coconut oil
- 1/2 cup raw honey
- 2 cups finely shredded coconut
- 1 cup large flake coconut
- 2 teaspoons of ground vanilla bean
- 1/2 cup chopped almonds or chia seeds (optional)
- 1/2 cup almond butter (optional)

Directions

a) Combine the coconut milk, coconut oil and cacao powder in a saucepan. Cook the mixture over medium heat, stirring until it comes to a boil and then boil for 1 minute.

b) Remove the mixture from the heat and stir in the shredded coconut, large flake coconut, raw honey and the vanilla. Add additional Ingredients if you want.

c) Spoon the mixture to a parchment lined baking sheet to cool.

48. Raw Brownies

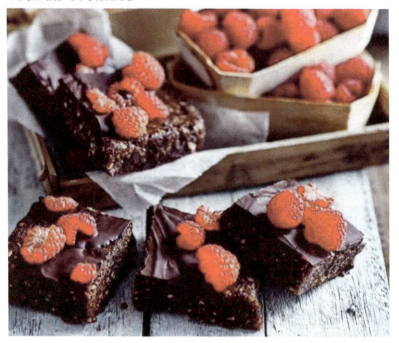

Ingredients

- 1 1/2 cups walnuts
- 1 cup pitted dates
- 1 1/2 teaspoons ground vanilla bean
- 1/3 cup unsweetened cocoa powder
- 1/3 cup almond butter

Directions

a) Add walnuts and salt to a food processor or blender. Mix until finely ground.

b) Add the vanilla, dates, and cocoa powder to the blender. Mix well and optionally add a couple drops of water at a time to make the mixture stick together.

c) Transfer the mixture into a pan and top with almond butter.

49. Ice cream

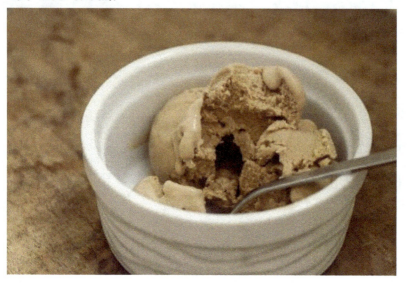

Directions

a) Freeze a banana cut into chunks and process it in blender once frozen and add half a teaspoons of cinnamon or 1 teaspoons of cocoa or both and eat it as ice-cream.

b) Other option would be to add one spoon of almond butter and mix it with mashed banana, it's also a delicious ice cream.

50. Apple Spice Cookies

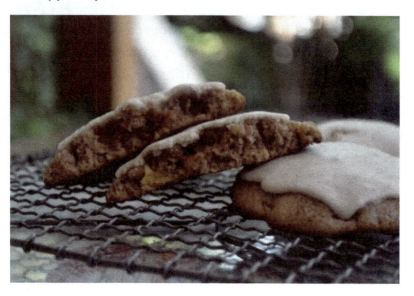

Ingredients

- 1 cup unsweetened almond butter
- 1/2 cup raw honey
- 1 egg and 1/2 teaspoons salt
- 1 apple, diced
- 1 teaspoons cinnamon
- 1/4 teaspoons ground cloves
- 1/8 teaspoons nutmeg
- 1 teaspoon fresh ginger, grated

Directions

a) heat oven to 350 degrees f. combine almond butter, egg, raw honey and salt in a bowl. add apple, spices, and ginger and stir. spoon batter onto a baking sheet 1 inches apart.

b) bake until set.

c) remove cookies and allow to cool on a cooling rack.

SOUPS

51. Cream of Broccoli Soup

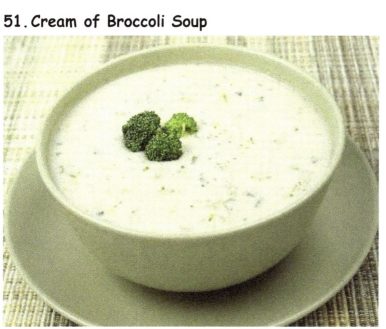

Serves 4

Ingredients

- 1 1/2 pounds broccoli, fresh
- 2 cups water
- 3/4 teaspoons salt, pepper to taste
- 1/2 cup tapioca flour, mixed with 1 cup cold water
- 1/2 cup coconut cream
- 1/2 cup low-fat farmers cheese

Directions

a) Steam or boil broccoli until it gets tender.

b) Put 2 cups water and coconut cream in top of double boiler.

c) Add salt, cheese and pepper. Heat until cheese gets melted.

d) Add broccoli. Mix water and tapioca flour in a small bowl.

e) Stir tapioca mixture into cheese mixture in double boiler and heat until soup thickens.

52. Lentil Soup

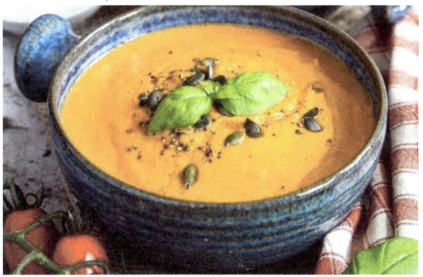

Serves 4-6

Ingredients

- 2 Tablespoons olive oil or avocado oil
- 1 cup finely chopped onion
- 1/2 cup chopped carrot
- 1/2 cup chopped celery
- 2 teaspoons salt
- 1 pound lentils
- 1 cup chopped tomatoes
- 2 quarts chicken or vegetable broth
- 1/2 teaspoons ground coriander and toasted cumin

Directions

a) Place the olive oil into a large Dutch oven. Set over medium heat. Once hot, add the celery, onion, carrot and salt and do until the onions are translucent.
b) Add the lentils, tomatoes, cumin, broth and coriander and stir to combine. Increase the heat and bring just to a boil.
c) Reduce the heat, cover and simmer at a low until the lentils are tender (approx. 35 to 40 minutes).
d) Puree with a bender to your preferred consistency (optional). Serve immediately.

53. Cold Cucumber Avocado Soup

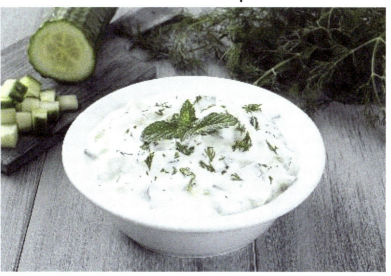

Serves 2-3

Ingredients

- 1 cucumber peeled, seeded and cut into 2-inch chunks
- 1 avocado, peeled
- 2 chopped scallions
- 1 cup chicken broth
- 3/4 cup Greek low-fat yogurt
- 2 Tablespoons lemon juice
- 1/2 teaspoons ground pepper, or to taste
- Chopped chives, dill, mint, scallions or cucumber

Directions

a) Combine the cucumber, avocado and scallions in a blender. Pulse until chopped.
b) Add yogurt, broth and lemon juice and continue until smooth.
c) Season with pepper and salt to taste and chill for 4 hours.
d) Taste for seasoning and garnish.

54. Gazpacho

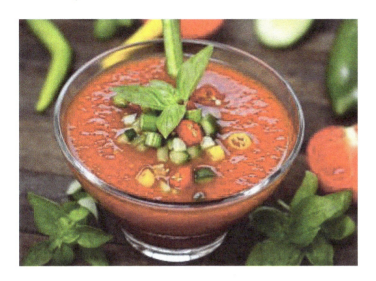

Serves 4

Ingredients

- 1/2 cup of flax seeds meal
- 1kg tomatoes, diced
- 1 red pepper and 1 green pepper, diced
- 1 cucumber, peeled and diced
- 2 cloves of garlic, peeled and crushed
- 150ml extra virgin olive oil or avocado oil
- 2 Tablespoons lemon juice
- Salt, to taste

Directions

a) Mix the peppers, tomatoes and cucumber with the crushed garlic and olive oil in the bowl of a blender.

b) Add flax meal to the mixture. Blend until smooth.

c) Add salt and lemon juice to taste and stir well.

d) Refrigerate until well chilled. Serve with black olives, hard-boiled egg, cilantro, mint or parsley.

55. Italian Beef Soup

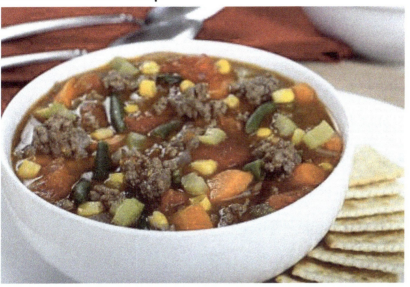

Serves 6

Ingredients

- 1 pound minced bee1 clove garlic, minced
- 2 cups beef broth
- few large tomatoes
- 1 cup sliced carrots
- 2 cups cooked beans
- 2 small zucchinis, cubed
- 2 cups spinach - rinsed and torn
- 1/4 teaspoons black pepper
- 1/4 teaspoons salt

Directions

a) Brown beef with garlic in a stockpot. Stir in broth, carrots and tomatoes. Season with salt and pepper.
b) Reduce heat, cover, and simmer for 15 minutes
c) Stir in beans with liquid and zucchini. Cover, and simmer until zucchini is tender.
d) Remove from heat, add spinach and cover. Serve after 5 minutes.

56. Creamy roasted mushroom

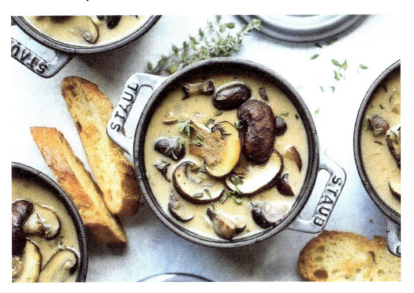

SERVES 4

Ingredients

- 1 pound Portobello mushrooms, cut into 1inch pieces
- 1/2-pound shiitake mushrooms, stemmed
- 6 Tablespoons olive oil or avocado oil
- 2 cups vegetable broth
- 1 1/2 Tablespoons coconut oil
- 1 onion, chopped
- 3 garlic cloves, minced
- 3 Tablespoons arrowroot flour
- 1 cup coconut cream
- 3/4 teaspoons chopped thyme

Directions

a) Heat oven to 400°F. Line one large baking sheets with foil. Spread mushrooms and drizzle some olive oil on them. Season with salt and pepper and toss. Cover with foil and bake them for half an hour. Uncover and continue baking 15 minutes more. Cool slightly. Mix one half of the mushrooms with one can of broth in a blender. Set aside.

b) Melt coconut oil in a large pot over high heat. Add onion and garlic and sauté until onion is translucent. Add flour and stir

2 minutes. Add cream, broth, and thyme. Stir in remaining cooked mushrooms and mushroom puree. Simmer over low heat until thickened (approx. 10 minutes). Season to taste with salt and pepper.

57. Black Bean Soup

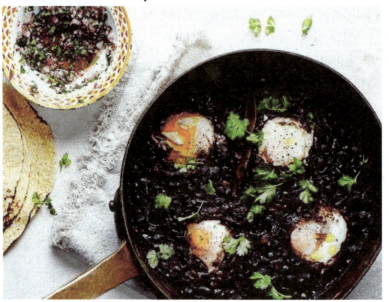

Serves 6-8
Ingredients

- 1/4 cup coconut oil
- 1/4 cup Onion, Diced
- 1/4 cup Carrots, Diced
- 1/4 cup Green Bell Pepper, Diced
- 1 cup beef broth
- 3 pounds cooked Black Beans
- 1 Tablespoons lemon juice
- 2 teaspoons Garlic
- 2 teaspoons Salt
- 1/2 teaspoons Black Pepper, Ground
- 2 teaspoons Chili Powder
- 8 oz. pork
- 1 Tablespoons tapioca flour
- 2 Tablespoons Water

Directions

a) Place coconut oil, onion, carrot, and bell pepper in a stock pot. Cook the veggies until tender. Bring broth to a boil.
b) Add cooked beans, broth and the remaining Ingredients (except tapioca flour and 2 Tablespoons water) to the

vegetables. Bring that mixture to a simmer and cook approximately 15 minutes.
c) Puree 1 quart of the soup in a blender and put back into the pot. Combine the tapioca flour and 2 Tablespoons water in a separate bowl.
d) Add the tapioca flour mixture to the bean soup and bring to a boil for 1 minute.

58. White Gazpacho

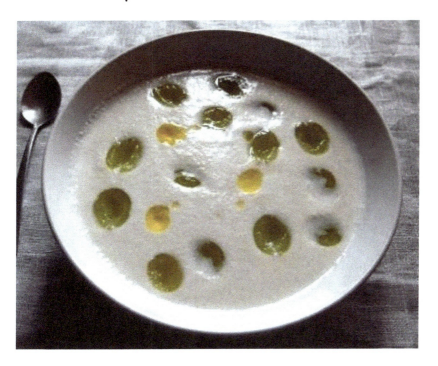

Serves 4-6

Ingredients

- 1 cup flax seeds meal
- 200 g almonds, blanched and skinned
- 3 cloves garlic
- 150 ml extra virgin olive oil or avocado oil
- 5 Tablespoons lemon juice
- 2 teaspoons salt
- 1-liter water
- 150 g grapes, seeded

Directions

a) Put flax meal with the almonds and garlic in the blender. Blend to a smooth paste. Add a little water if necessary. Add the oil in a slow stream with the motor running. Add the lemon juice and salt too.

b) Pour the mixture into a pitcher and add the remaining water. Add salt or lemon juice to taste. Chill the soup.

c) Stir before serving and garnish with grapes.

59. Squash soup

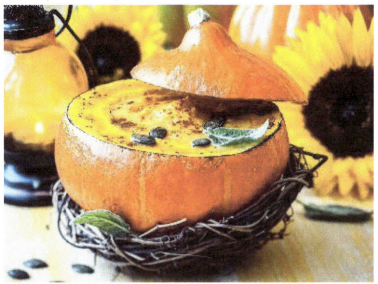

Serves 4-6

Ingredients
- 1 Squash
- 1 carrot, chopped
- 1 onion (diced)
- 3/4 - 1 cup coconut milk
- 1/4 - 1/2 cup water
- olive oil or avocado oil
- Salt
- Pepper
- Cinnamon
- Turmeric

Directions

a) Cut the squash and spoon out the seeds. Cut it into large pieces and place on a baking sheet. Sprinkle with salt, olive oil, and pepper and bake at 375 degrees F until soft (approx. 1 hour). Let cool.

b) In the meantime, sauté the onions in olive oil (put it in a soup pot). Add the carrots. Add 3/4 cup coconut milk and 1/4 cup water after few minutes and let simmer. Scoop the squash out of its skin. Add it to the soup pot. Stir to combine the ingredients and let simmer a few minutes. Add more milk or water if needed. Season to taste with the salt, pepper and spices. Blend until smooth and creamy.

c) Sprinkle it with toasted pumpkin seeds.

60. Kale White Bean Pork Soup

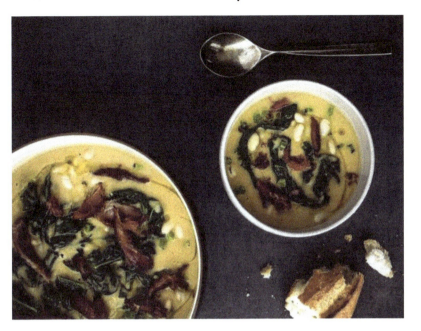

SERVES 4-6

Ingredients

- 2 Tablespoons each extra-virgin olive oil
- 3 Tablespoons chili powder
- 1 Tablespoons jalapeno hot sauce
- 2 pounds bone-in pork chops
- Salt
- 4 stalks celery, chopped
- 1 large white onion, chopped
- 3 cloves garlic, chopped
- 2 cups chicken broth
- 2 cups diced tomatoes
- 2 cups cooked white beans
- 6 cups packed Kale

Directions

a) Preheat the broiler. Whisk hot sauce, 1 Tablespoons olive oil and chili powder in a bowl. Season the pork chops with 1/2 teaspoons salt. Rub chops with the spice mixture on both sides and place them on a rack set over a baking sheet. Set aside.

b) Heat 1 Tablespoons coconut oil in a large pot over high heat. Add the celery, garlic, onion and the remaining 2 Tablespoons chili powder. Cook until onions are translucent, stirring (approx. 8 minutes).

c) Add tomatoes and the chicken broth to the pot. Cook and stir occasionally until reduced by about one-third (approx. 7 minutes). Add the kale and the beans. Reduce the heat to medium, cover and cook until the kale is tender (approx. 7 minutes). Add up to 1/2 cup water if the mixture looks dry and season with salt.

d) In the meantime, broil the pork until browned

61. Greek lemon chicken soup

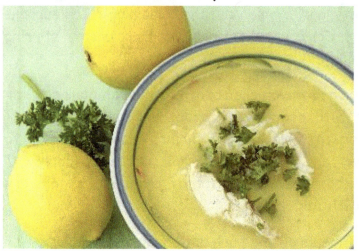

Serves 4

Ingredients
- 4 cups chicken broth
- 1/4 cup uncooked quinoa
- salt and pepper
- 3 eggs
- 3 Tablespoons lemon juice
- Handful fresh dill (chopped)
- shredded roasted chicken (optional)

Directions

a) Bring the broth to a boil in a saucepan. Add the quinoa and cook until tender. Season with the salt and pepper. Reduce heat to low and let simmer. In a separate bowl, whisk lemon juice and the eggs until smooth. Add about 1 cup of the hot broth into the egg/lemon mixture and whisk to combine.

b) Add the mixture back to the saucepan. Stir until the soup becomes opaque and thickens. Add dill, salt and pepper to taste and chicken if you have it, and serve.

62. Egg-Drop Soup

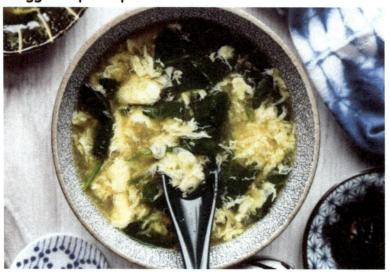

SERVES 4-6

Ingredients

- 1 1/2 quarts chicken broth
- 2 Tablespoons Tapioca flour, mixed in 1/4 cup cold water
- 2 eggs, slightly beaten with a fork
- 2 scallions, chopped, including green ends

Directions

a) Bring broth to a boil. Slowly pour in the tapioca flour mixture while stirring the broth. The broth should thicken.

b) Reduce heat and let it simmer. Mix in the eggs very slowly while stirring.

c) As soon as the last drop of egg is in, turn off the heat.

d) Serve with chopped scallions on top.

63. Creamy Tomato Basil Soup

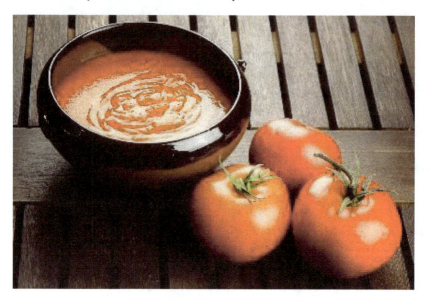

SERVES 6

Ingredients

- 4 tomatoes - peeled, seeded and diced
- 4 cups tomato juice
- 14 leaves fresh basil
- 1 cup coconut cream
- salt to taste
- ground black pepper to taste

Directions

a) Combine tomatoes and tomato juice in stock pot. Simmer 30 minutes.
b) Puree mixture with basil leaves in a processor.
c) Put back in a stock pot and add coconut cream.
d) Add salt and pepper to taste.

MAIN DISH

64. Lentil Stew

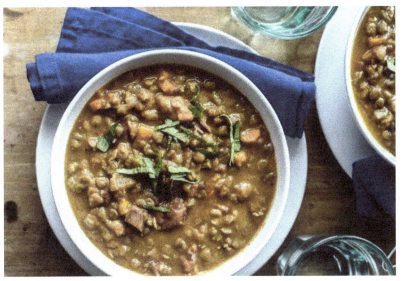

Ingredients

- 1 cup dry lentils
- 3 1/2 cups chicken broth
- few tomatoes
- 1 medium potato chopped + 1/2 cup chopped carrot
- 1/2 cup chopped onion + 1/2 cup chopped celery (optional)
- few sprigs of parsley and basil + 1 garlic clove (minced)
- 1 pound of cubed lean pork or beef + pepper to taste

Directions

a) You can eat a salad of your choice with this stew.

65. Braised Green Peas with Beef

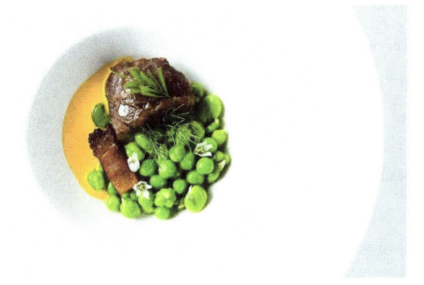

SERVES 1

Ingredients

- 1 cup fresh or frozen green peas
- 1 onion, finely chopped
- 2 cloves of garlic, thinly sliced and 1/2 inch of peeled/sliced fresh ginger (if you like)
- 1/2 teaspoons red pepper flakes, or to taste
- 1 tomato, roughly chopped
- 1 chopped carrot
- 1 Tablespoons coconut oil
- 1/2 cup chicken broth
- 4 oz. cubed beef
- Salt and freshly ground black pepper

Directions

a) Heat the coconut oil in a skillet over medium heat.

b) Sauté the onion, garlic and ginger until they are soft. Add the red pepper, carrot, and tomatoes and sauté until the tomato begins to soften. Add in the green peas. Add 4 oz. cubed lean beef.

c) Add in the broth and simmer over medium heat. Cover and cook until the peas are tender. Season to taste with salt and pepper.

66. White Chicken Chili

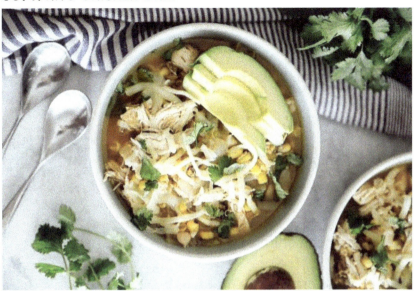

SERVES: 5

Ingredients

- 4 large boneless, skinless chicken breasts
- 2 green bell peppers
- 1 large yellow onion
- 1 jalapeno
- 1/2 cup diced green chilies (optional)
- 1/2 cup of spring onions
- 1.5 Tablespoons coconut oil
- 3 cups cooked white beans
- 3.5 cups chicken or vegetable broth
- 1 teaspoons ground cumin
- 1/4 teaspoons cayenne pepper
- salt to taste

Directions

a) Bring a pot of water to boil. Add the chicken breasts and cook until cooked through. Drain water and allow chicken to cool. When cool, shred and set aside.

b) Dice the bell peppers, jalapeno and onion. Melt the coconut oil in a pot over high heat. Add the peppers and onions and sauté until soft, approx. 8-10 minutes.

c) Add the broth, beans, chicken and spices to the pot. Stir and bring to a low boil. Cover and simmer for 25-30 minutes.

d) Simmer for 10 more minutes and stir occasionally. Remove from heat. Let stand for 10 minutes to thicken. Top with cilantro.

67. Kale Pork

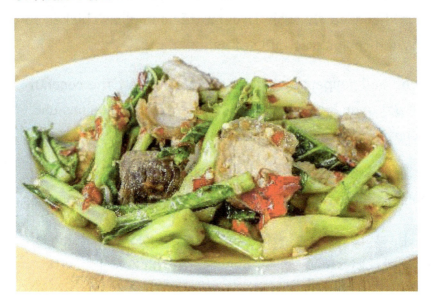

SERVES 4

Ingredients

- 1 Tablespoons coconut oil
- 1-pound pork tenderloin, trimmed and cut into 1-inch pieces
- 3/4 teaspoons salt
- 1 medium onion, finely chopped
- 4 cloves garlic, minced
- 2 teaspoons paprika
- 1/4 teaspoons crushed red pepper (optional)
- 1 cup white wine
- 4 plum tomatoes, chopped
- 4 cups chicken broth
- 1 bunch kale, chopped
- 2 cups cooked white beans

Directions

a) Heat coconut oil in a pot over medium heat. Add pork, season with salt and cook until no longer pink. Transfer to a plate and leave juices in the pot.

b) Add onion to the pot and cook until turns translucent. Add paprika, garlic and crushed red pepper and cook about 30 seconds. Add tomatoes and wine, increase heat and stir to scrape up any browned bits. Add broth. Bring to a boil.

c) Add kale and stir until it wilts. Lower the heat and simmer, until the kale is tender. Stir in beans, pork and pork juices. Simmer for 2 more minutes.

68. Squash Cauliflower Curry

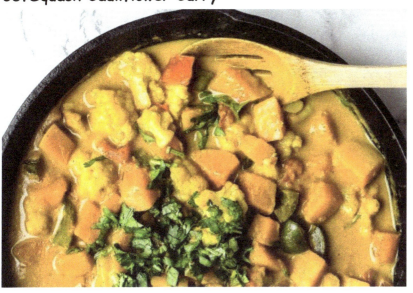

Serves: 6

Ingredients

- 3 cups peeled, chopped squash
- 2 cups thick coconut milk
- 3 Tablespoons coconut oil
- 2 Tablespoons raw honey
- 2 pounds tomatoes
- 1 and 1/4 cup brown rice, uncooked
- 1 cup chopped Cauliflower
- 1 cup chopped Green Peppers
- Cilantro for topping

Directions

a) Cook brown rice. Set aside.

b) Make Curry Paste. Pour the coconut milk into the skillet and mix the curry and raw honey into the coconut milk. Add the cauliflower, squash, and green peppers. Cover and simmer until squash is tender. Remove from heat and let stand for 10 minutes. The sauce will thicken.

c) Serve the curry over brown rice. Add chopped cilantro before serving.

69. Crockpot Red Curry Lamb

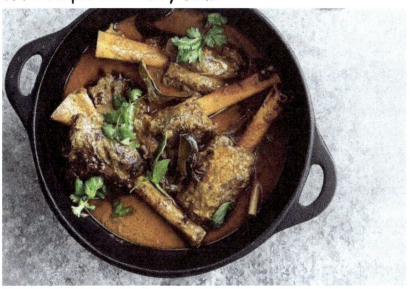

Serves: 16

Ingredients

- 3 pounds cubed lamb meat
- Curry Paste
- 4 cups tomato paste
- 1 teaspoons salt plus more to taste
- 1/2 cup coconut milk or cream

Directions

a) Make the Curry Paste. Add lamb and the curry paste in a crockpot. Pour one cup of tomato paste over the lamb. Add 2 cups of water to the crockpot. Stir, cover and cook on high for 2 hours or low for 4-5 hours. Taste and season with salt.

b) Stir in the coconut milk and sprinkle with cilantro before serving. Serve over brown rice or naan bread.

70. Easy Lentil Dhal

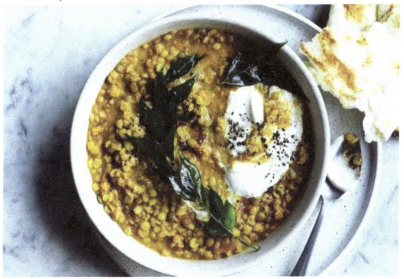

SERVES: 6

Ingredients

- 2 1/2 cups lentils
- 5-6 cups of water
- Curry Paste
- 1/2 cup coconut milk
- 1/3 cup water
- 1/2 teaspoons salt + 1/4 teaspoons black pepper
- lime juice
- Cilantro and spring onions for garnish

Directions

a) Bring the water to a boil in a large pot. Add lentils and cook uncovered for 10 minutes, stirring frequently.

b) Remove from heat. Stir in remaining Ingredients.

c) Season with salt and herbs for garnish.

71. Gumbo

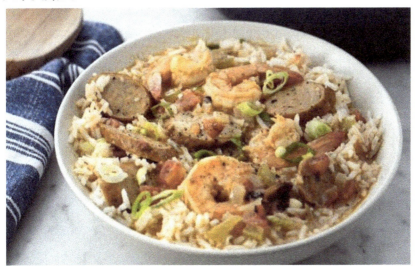

Ingredients

- 1-pound medium shrimp peeled
- 1/2 pound skinless, boneless chicken breasts
- 1/2 cup coconut oil
- 3/4 cup almond flour
- 2 cups chopped onions
- 1 cup chopped celery
- 1 cup chopped green pepper
- 1 teaspoons ground cumin
- 1 Tablespoons minced fresh garlic
- 1 teaspoon fresh thyme chopped
- 1/2 teaspoons red pepper
- 6 cups chicken broth
- 2 cups diced tomatoes
- 3 cups sliced okra
- 1/2 cup fresh parsley chopped
- 2 bay leaves
- 1 teaspoon hot sauce

Directions

a) Sauté' chicken on high heat until brown in a large pot. Remove and set aside. Chop onions, celery, and green pepper and set aside.

b) Place oil and flour in pot. Stir well and brown to make a roux. When roux is done add chopped vegetables. Sauté on low heat for 10 minutes.

c) Slowly add chicken broth stirring constantly.

d) Add chicken and all other Ingredients except the okra, shrimp and parsley, which will be saved for the end.

e) Cover and simmer on low for half an hour. Remove lid and cook for half an hour more, stirring occasionally.

f) Add shrimp, okra and parsley. Continue to cook on low heat uncovered for 15 minutes.

72. Chickpea Curry

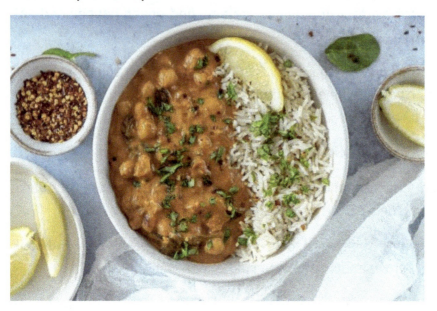

SERVES 4

Ingredients

- Curry Paste
- 4 cups cooked chickpeas
- 1 cup chopped cilantro

Directions

a) Make Curry Paste. Mix in chickpeas and their liquid.
b) Continue to cook. Stir until all ingredients are blended.
c) Remove from heat. Stir in cilantro just before serving, reserving 1 Tablespoons for garnish.

73. Red Curry Chicken

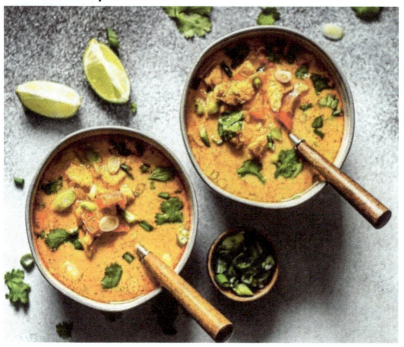

SERVES: 6

Ingredients

- 2 cups cubed chicken meat
- Curry Paste
- 2 cups tomato paste
- 1/4 cup coconut milk or cream
- Cilantro for garnishing
- Brown rice for serving

Directions

a) Make Curry Paste. Add the tomato paste; stir and simmer until smooth. Add the chicken and the cream.

b) Stir to combine and simmer for 15-20 minutes.

c) Serve with brown rice and cilantro.

74. Braised Green Beans with Pork

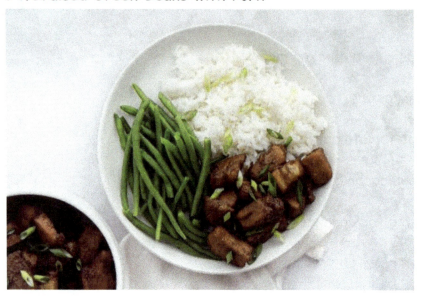

Serves 1

Ingredients

- 1cup fresh or frozen green beans
- 1 onion, finely chopped
- 2 cloves of garlic, thinly sliced
- 1/2 inch of peeled/sliced fresh ginger
- 1/2 teaspoons red pepper flakes, or to taste
- 1 tomato, roughly chopped
- 1 Tablespoons coconut oil
- 1/2 cup chicken broth
- Salt and ground black pepper
- 1/4 lemon, cut into wedges, to serve
- 5 oz. lean pork

Directions

a) Cut each bean in half. Heat the coconut oil in a skillet over medium heat. Sauté the onion, garlic and ginger over medium heat until they are soft.

b) Add the red pepper and tomatoes and sauté until the tomato begins to break down. Stir in the green beans. Add 5 oz. cubed lean pork.

c) Add broth and bring to a simmer over medium heat. Cover and cook until the beans are tender.

d) Season to taste with salt and pepper. Serve with lemon wedge on the side.

75. Ratatouille

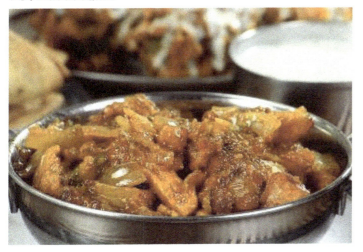

Serves 4-6
Ingredients

- 2 large eggplants
- 3 medium zucchinis
- 2 medium onions
- 2 red or green peppers
- 4 large tomatoes
- 2 cloves garlic, crushed
- 4 Tablespoons coconut oil
- 1 Tablespoons fresh basil
- Salt and freshly milled black pepper

Directions

a) Cut eggplant and zucchini into 1 inch slices. Then cut each slice in half. Salt them and leave them for one hour. The salt will draw out the bitterness.

b) Chop peppers and onions. Skin the tomatoes by boiling them for few minutes. Then quarter them, take out the seeds and chop the flesh. Fry garlic and the onions in the coconut oil in a saucepan for a 10 minutes. Add the peppers. Dry the eggplant and zucchini and add them to the saucepan. Add the basil, salt and pepper. Stir and simmer for half an hour.

c) Add the tomato flesh, check the seasoning and cook for an additional 15 minutes with the lid off.

76. Barbecued Beef

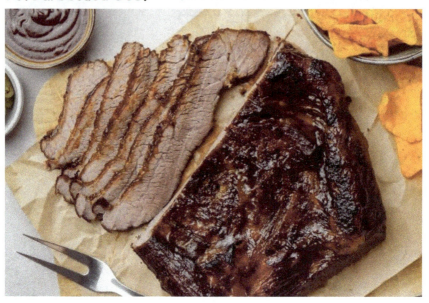

Serves 8

Ingredients

- 1-1/2 cups tomato paste
- 1/4 cup lemon juice
- 2 Tablespoons Mustard
- 1/2 teaspoons salt
- 1 chopped carrot
- 1/4 teaspoons ground black pepper
- 1/2 teaspoons minced garlic
- 4 pounds boneless chuck roast

Directions

a) In a large bowl, combine tomato paste, lemon juice and mustard. Stir in salt, pepper and garlic.

b) Place chuck roast and carrot in a slow cooker. Pour tomato mixture over chuck roast. Cover, and cook on low for 7 to 9 hours.

c) Remove chuck roast from slow cooker, shred with a fork, and return to the slow cooker. Stir meat to evenly coat with sauce. Continue cooking approximately 1 hour.

77. Beef Tenderloin with Shallots

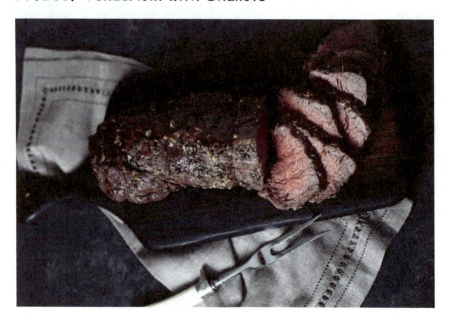

Ingredients

- 3/4 pound shallots, halved lengthwise
- 1-1/2 Tablespoons olive oil or avocado oil
- salt and pepper to taste
- 3 cups beef broth
- 3/4 cup red wine
- 1-1/2 teaspoons tomato paste
- 2 pounds beef tenderloin roast, trimmed
- 1 teaspoons dried thyme
- 3 Tablespoons coconut oil
- 1 Tablespoons almond flour

Directions

a) Heat oven to 375 degrees F. Toss shallots with olive oil to coat in a baking pan and season with salt and pepper. Roast until shallots are tender, stirring occasionally, about half an hour.

b) Combine wine and beef broth in a sauce pan and bring to a boil. Cook over high heat. Volume should be reduced by half. Add in tomato paste. Set aside.

c) Pat beef dry and sprinkle with salt and thyme and pepper. Add beef to pan oiled with coconut oil. Brown on all sides over high heat.

d) Put pan back to the oven. Roast beef about half an hour for medium rare. Transfer beef to platter. Cover loosely with foil.

e) Place pan on stove top and add broth mixture. Bring to boil and stir to scrape up any browned bits. Transfer to a different saucepan, and bring to simmer. Mix 1 1/2 Tablespoons coconut oil and flour in small bowl and mix. Whisk into broth, and simmer until sauce thickens. Stir in roasted shallots. Season with salt and pepper.

f) Cut beef into 1/2-inch-thick slices. Spoon some sauce over.

78. Chili

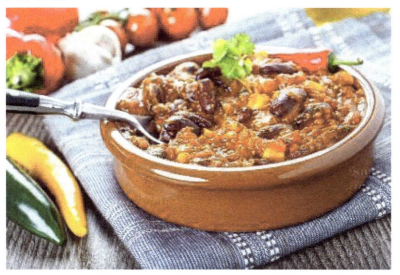

Ingredients

- 2 Tablespoons coconut oil
- 2 onions, chopped
- 3 cloves garlic, minced
- 1-pound ground beef
- 3/4-pound beef sirloin, cubed
- 2cups diced tomatoes
- 1 cup strong brewed coffee
- 1 cup tomato paste
- 2 cups beef broth
- 1 Tablespoons cumin seeds
- 1 Tablespoons unsweetened cocoa powder
- 1 teaspoons dried oregano
- 1 teaspoons ground cayenne pepper
- 1 teaspoons ground coriander
- 1 teaspoons salt
- 6 cups cooked kidney beans
- 4 fresh hot chili peppers, chopped

Directions

a) Heat oil in a saucepan over medium heat. Cook garlic, onions, sirloin and ground beef in oil until the meat is browned and the onions are translucent.

b) Mix in the diced tomatoes, coffee, tomato paste and beef broth. Season with oregano, cumin, cocoa powder, cayenne pepper, coriander and salt. Stir in hot chile peppers and 3 cups of the beans. Reduce heat to low, and simmer for two hours.

c) Stir in the 3 remaining cups of beans. Simmer for another 30 minutes.

79. Glazed Meatloaf

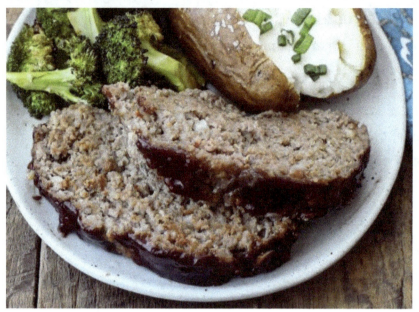

Serves 4

Ingredients

- 1/2 cup tomato paste
- 1/4 cup lemon juice, divided
- 1 teaspoons mustard powder
- 2 pounds ground beef
- 1 cup flax seeds meal
- 1/4 cup chopped onion
- 1 egg, beaten

Directions

a) Heat oven to 350 degrees F. Combine mustard, tomato paste, 1 Tablespoons lemon juice in a small bowl.

b) Combine onion, ground beef, flax, egg and remaining lemon juice in a separate larger bowl.

c) And add 1/3 of the tomato paste mixture from the smaller bowl. Mix all well and place in a loaf pan.

d) Bake at 350 degrees F for one hour. Drain any excess fat and coat with remaining tomato paste mixture. Bake for 10 more minutes.

80. Eggplant Lasagna

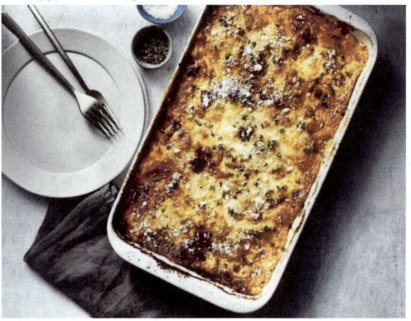

Serves 4-6

Ingredients

- 2 large eggplants, peeled and sliced lengthwise into strips
- coconut oil
- salt and pepper

Meat Sauce

- 2 cups low-fat farmers cheese
- 2 eggs
- 3 green onions, chopped
- 1 cup shredded low-fat mozzarella cheese

Directions

a) Heat oven to 425 degrees.

b) Oil cookie sheet and arrange eggplant slice. Sprinkle with salt and pepper. Bake slices 5 minutes on each side. Lower oven temp to 375.

c) Brown onion, meat and garlic in coconut oil for 5 minutes. Add mushrooms and red pepper, and cook for 5 minutes. Add tomatoes, spinach and spices and simmer for 5-10 minutes.

d) Blend farmers' cheese, egg and onion mixture. Spread one third of meat sauce in bottom of a glass pan. Layer one half of eggplant slices and one half farmers' cheese. Repeat. Add last layer of sauce and then mozzarella on top.

e) Cover with foil. Bake at 375 degrees for one hour. Remove foil and bake until cheese is browned. Let it rest 10 minutes before serving.

81. Stuffed Eggplant

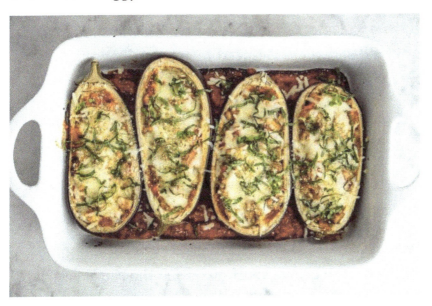

Directions

a) Rinse the eggplants. Cut off a slice from one end. Make a wide slit and salt them. De-seed tomatoes. Chop them finely.

b) Cut the onions in thin slices. Chop the garlic cloves. Place them in a frying pan with coconut oil.

c) Add the tomatoes, salt parsley, cumin, pepper, hot peppers and ground beef. Sauté for 10 minutes.

d) Squeeze eggplants, so the bitter juice goes out. Fill the wide slit with the ground beef mix. Pour the remaining mix over. Heat the oven to 375F in the meantime.

e) Place eggplants a baking pan. Sprinkle them with olive oil, lemon juice and 1 cup of water.

f) Cover the pan with a foil.

82. Stuffed Red Peppers with Beef

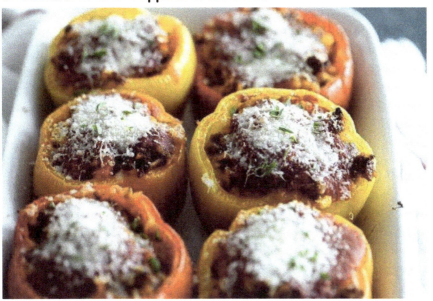

Ingredients

- 6 red bell peppers
- salt to taste
- 1-pound ground beef
- 1/3 cup chopped onion
- salt and pepper to taste
- 2 cups chopped tomatoes
- 1/2 cup uncooked brown rice or
- 1/2 cup water
- 2 cups tomato soup
- water as needed

Directions

a) Cook peppers in boiling water for 5 minutes and drain.

b) Sprinkle salt inside each pepper, and set aside.
In a skillet, sauté onions and beef until beef is browned. Drain off excess fat. Season with salt and pepper. Stir in rice, tomatoes and 1/2 cup water. Cover, and simmer until rice is tender. Remove from heat. Stir in the cheese.

c) Heat the oven to 350 degrees F. Stuff each pepper with the rice and beef mixture. Place peppers open side up in a baking dish. Combine tomato soup with just enough water to make the soup a gravy consistency in a separate bowl.

d) Pour over the peppers.

e) Bake covered for 25 to 35 minutes.

83. Super Goulash

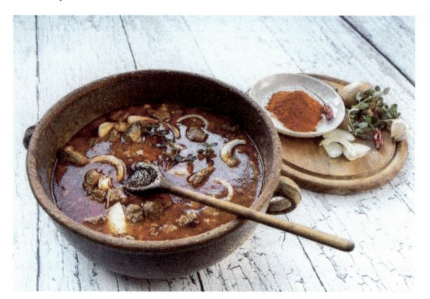

SERVES 4-6

Ingredients

- 3 cups cauliflower
- 1-pound ground beef
- 1 medium onion, chopped
- salt to taste
- ground black pepper to taste
- garlic to taste
- 2 cups cooked kidney beans
- 1 cup tomato paste

Directions

a) Brown the ground beef and onion in a skillet, over medium heat. Drain off the fat. Add garlic, salt and pepper to taste.

b) Stir in the cauliflower, kidney beans and tomato paste. Cook until cauliflower is done.

84. Frijoles Charros

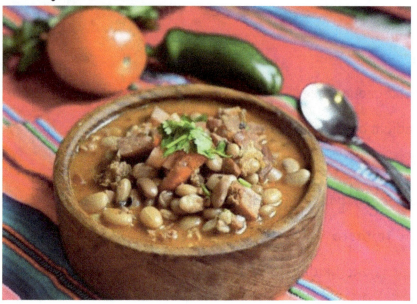

Serves 4-6

Ingredients

- 1-pound dry pinto beans
- 5 cloves garlic, chopped
- 1 teaspoons salt
- 1/2-pound pork, diced
- 1 onion, chopped and 2 fresh tomatoes, diced
- few sliced sliced jalapeno peppers
- 1/3 cup chopped cilantro

Directions

a) Place pinto beans in a slow cooker. Cover with water. Mix in garlic and salt. Cover, and cook 1 hour on High.

b) Cook the pork in a skillet over high heat until brown. Drain the fat. Place onion in the skillet. Cook until tender. Mix in jalapenos and tomatoes. Cook until heated through. Transfer to the slow cooker and stir into the beans. Continue cooking for 4 hours on Low. Mix in cilantro about half an hour before the end of the cook time.

85. Chicken Cacciatore

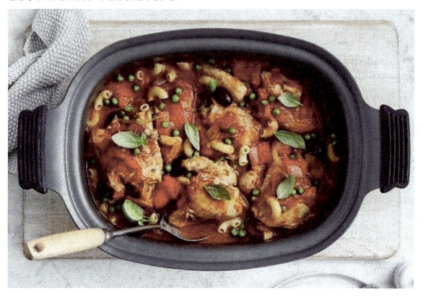

Serves 8
Ingredients

- 4 pounds of chicken thighs, with skin on
- 2 Tablespoons extra virgin olive oil or avocado oil
- Salt
- 1 sliced onion
- 1/3 cup red wine
- 1 sliced red or green bell pepper
- 8 ounces sliced cremini mushrooms
- 2 sliced garlic cloves
- 3 cups peeled and chopped tomatoes
- 1/2 teaspoons ground black pepper
- 1 teaspoon dry oregano
- 1 teaspoon dry thyme
- 1 sprig fresh rosemary
- 1 Tablespoons fresh parsley

Directions

a) Pat the chicken on all sides with salt. Heat the olive oil in a skillet on medium. Brown few chicken pieces skin side down in the pan (don't overcrowd) for 5 minutes, then turn. Set aside. Make sure you have 2 Tablespoons of the rendered fat left.

b) Add the onions, mushrooms and bell peppers to the pan. Increase the heat to medium high. Cook until the onions are tender, stirring, about 10 minutes. Add the garlic and cook a minute more.

c) Add the wine. Scrape up any browned bits and simmer until the wine is reduced by half. Add the tomatoes, pepper, oregano, thyme and a teaspoons of salt. Simmer uncovered for maybe 5 more minutes. Put the chicken pieces on top of the tomatoes, skin side up. Lower the heat. Cover the skillet with the lid slightly ajar.

d) Cook the chicken on a low simmer. Turning and baste from time to time. Add rosemary and cook until the meat is tender, about 30 to 40 minutes. Garnish with parsley.

86. Cabbage Stewed with Meat

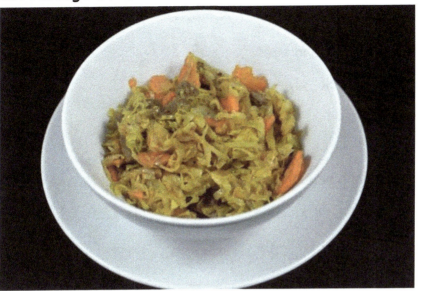

Serves 8

Ingredients

- 1-1/2 pounds ground beef
- 1 cup beef stock
- 1 chopped onion
- 1 bay leaf
- 1/4 teaspoons pepper
- 2 sliced celery ribs
- 4 cups shredded cabbage
- 1 carrot, sliced
- 1 cup tomato paste
- 1/4 teaspoons salt

Directions

a) Brown ground meat in a pot. Add beef stock, onion, pepper and bay leaf. Cover and simmer until tender (about 30 minutes). Add celery, cabbage and carrot.

b) Cover and simmer until vegetables are tender. Mix in tomato paste and seasoning blend. Simmer uncovered for 20 minutes.

87. Beef Stew with Peas and Carrots

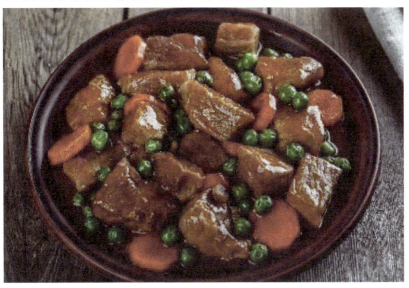

Serves 8
Ingredients

- 1-1/2 cups chopped carrots·
- 1 cup chopped onions
- 2 Tablespoons coconut oil
- 1-1/2 cups green peas
- 4 cups beef stock
- 1/2 teaspoons Salt
- 1/4 teaspoons ground black pepper
- 1/2 teaspoons minced garlic
- 4 pounds boneless chuck roast

Directions

a) Cook the onions in coconut oil on medium until they are tender (few minutes). Add all other Ingredients and stir.

b) Cover and cook on low heat for 2 hours. Mix almond flour with some cold water, add to the stew and cook for another minute.

88. Green Chicken Stew

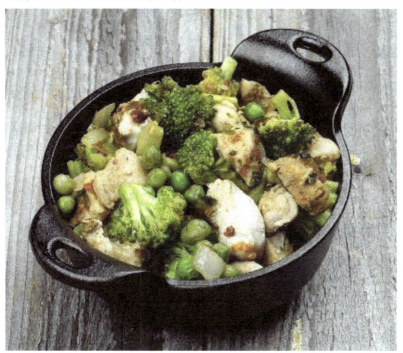

Serves 6-8

Ingredients

- 1-1/2 cups broccoli florets
- 1 cup chopped celery stalks
- 1 cup sliced leeks
- 2 Tablespoons coconut oil
- 1-1/2 cups green peas
- 2 cups chicken stock
- 1/2 teaspoons Salt
- 1/4 teaspoons ground black pepper
- 1/2 teaspoons minced garlic

- 4 pounds boneless skinless chicken pieces

Directions

a) Cook the leeks in coconut oil on medium until they are tender (few minutes). Add all other Ingredients and stir.

b) Cover and cook on low heat for 1 hour. Mix almond flour with some cold water, add to the stew and cook for another minute.

89. Irish Stew

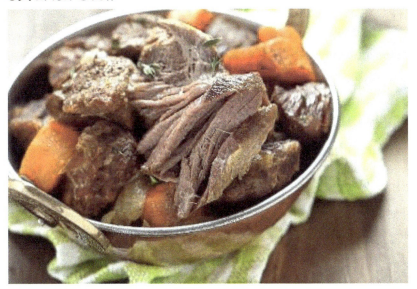

Serves 8
Ingredients

- 2 chopped onions
- 2 Tablespoons coconut oil
- 1 sprig dried thyme
- 2 1/2 pounds chopped meat from lamb neck
- 6 chopped carrots
- 2 Tablespoons brown rice
- 5 cups chicken stock
- Salt
- Ground black pepper
- 1 bouquet garni (thyme, parsley and bay leaf)
- 2 chopped sweet potatoes
- 1 bunch chopped parsley
- 1 bunch chives

Directions

a) Cook the onions in coconut oil on medium until they are tender. Add the dried thyme and lamb and stir. Add brown rice, carrots and chicken stock. Add salt, pepper and bouquet garni. Cover and cook on low heat for 2 hours. Place sweet potatoes on top of the stew and cook for 30 minutes until the meat is falling apart.

b) Garnish with parsley and chives.

90. Hungarian Pea Stew

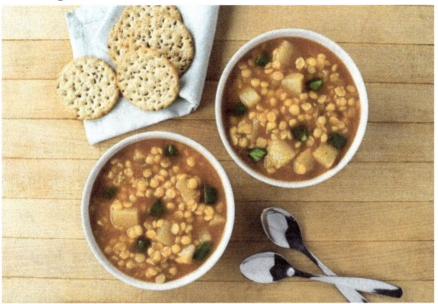

Serves 8
Ingredients

- 6 cups green peas
- 1 pound cubed pork
- 2 Tablespoons olive oil or avocado oil
- 3 1/2 Tablespoons almond flour
- 2 Tablespoons chopped parsley
- 1 cup water
- 1/2 teaspoons salt
- 1 cup coconut milk
- 1 teaspoons coconut sugar

Directions

a) Simmer the pork and green peas in the olive oil over medium heat until almost tender (approx. 10 minutes)

b) Add salt, chopped parsley, coconut sugar and almond flour, and cook for another minute.

c) Add water then milk and stir.

d) Cook for another 4 minutes over low heat, stirring occasionally.

91. Chicken Tikka Masala

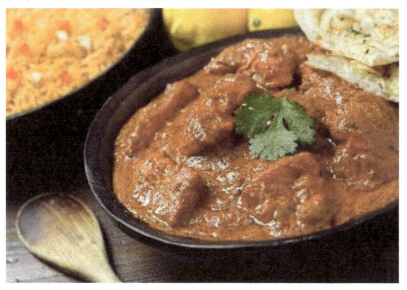

Ingredients

- 5 pounds chicken pieces, skinless, bone in
- 3 Tablespoons toasted paprika
- 2 Tablespoons toasted ground coriander seed
- 12 chopped cloves garlic
- 3 Tablespoons chopped fresh ginger
- 2 cups yogurt
- 3/4 cup lemon juice (4 to 6 lemons)
- 1 teaspoons sea salt
- 4 Tablespoons coconut oil
- 1 sliced onion
- 4 cups chopped tomatoes
- 1/2 cup chopped cilantro
- 1 cup coconut cream

Directions

a) Score chicken deeply at 1-inch intervals with a knife. Place chicken in a large baking dish.

b) Combine coriander, cumin, paprika, turmeric, and cayenne in a bowl and mix. Set aside 3 Tablespoons of this spice mixture. Combine remaining 6 Tablespoons spice mixture with 8 cloves garlic garlic, yogurt, 2 Tablespoons ginger, 1/4 cup salt and 1/2 cup lemon juice in a large bowl and combine. Pour marinade over chicken pieces.

c) Heat coconut oil in a large pot over medium-high heat and add remaining garlic and ginger. Add onions. Cook about 10 minutes, stirring occasionally. Add reserved spice mixture and cook until fragrant, about half a minute. Scrape up any browned bits from bottom of pan and add tomatoes and half of cilantro. Simmer for 15 minutes. Let cool slightly and puree.

d) Stir in coconut cream and remaining one quarter cup lemon juice. Season to taste with salt and set aside until chicken is cooked.

e) Cook chicken on a grill or under a broiler.

f) Remove chicken from bone and cut into rough bite-sized chunks. Add chicken chunks to pot of sauce. Bring to a simmer over medium heat and cook about 10 minutes.

92. Greek Beef Stew (Stifado)

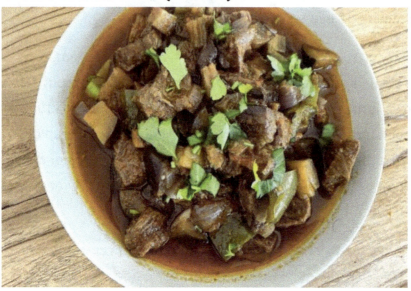

Serves 8

Ingredients

- 4 large pieces of veal or beef osso bucco
- 20 whole shallots, peeled
- 3 bay leaves
- 8 garlic cloves
- 3 sprigs rosemary
- 6 whole pimento
- 5 whole cloves
- 1/2 teaspoons ground nutmeg

- 1/2 cup olive oil or avocado oil
- 1/3 cup apple cider vinegar
- 1 Tablespoons salt
- 2 cups tomato paste
- 1/4 teaspoons black pepper

Directions

a) Mix vinegar and tomato paste and set aside. Place the meat, shallots, garlic and all spices in the pot.

b) Add the tomato paste, oil and vinegar. Cover the pot, bring to low boil and simmer on low for 2 hours. Do not open and stir, just shake the pot occasionally.

c) Serve with brown rice or maybe quinoa.

93. Meat Stew with Red Beans

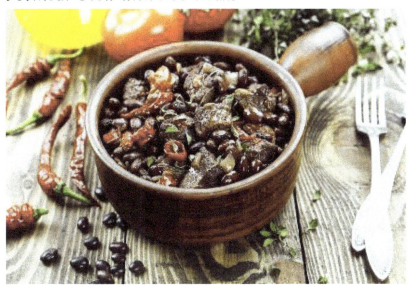

Serves 8

Ingredients

- 3 Tablespoons olive oil or avocado oil
- 1/2 chopped onion
- 1 lb. lean cubed stewing beef
- 2 teaspoons ground cumin
- 2 teaspoons ground turmeric (optional)
- 1/2 teaspoons ground cinnamon (optional)
- 2 1/2 cups water
- 5 Tablespoons chopped fresh parsley
- 3 Tablespoons snipped chives
- 2 cups cooked kidney beans
- 1 lemon, juice of
- 1 Tablespoons almond flour
- salt and black pepper

Directions

a) Sauté the onion in a pan with two tablespoons of the oil until tender.

b) Add beef and cook until meat is browned on all sides. Stir in turmeric, cinnamon (both optional) and cumin and cook for one minute. Add water and bring to a boil.

c) Cover and simmer over low heat for 45 minutes. Stir occasionally. Sauté parsley and chives with the remaining 1 Tablespoons of olive oil for about 2 minutes and add this mixture to the beef. Add kidney beans and lemon juice and season with salt and pepper.

d) Stir in one Tablespoons of almond flour mixed with a bit of water to thicken the stew. Simmer uncovered for half an hour until meat gets tender. Serve with brown rice.

94. Lamb and Sweet Potato Stew

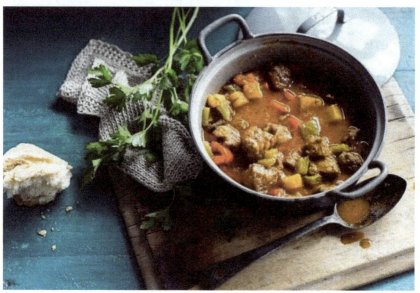

Serves 8

Ingredients

- 1-1/2 cups tomato paste
- 1/4 cup lemon juice
- 2 Tablespoons Mustard
- 1/2 teaspoons Salt
- 1/4 teaspoons ground black pepper
- 1/4 cup chunky almond butter
- 2 cubed sweet potatoes
- 1/2 teaspoons minced garlic
- 4 pounds boneless chuck roast

Directions

a) In a large bowl, combine tomato paste, lemon juice, almond butter and mustard. Stir in salt, pepper, garlic and cubed sweet potato.
 Place chuck roast in a slow cooker. Pour tomato mixture over chuck roast.

b) Cover, and cook on low for 7 to 9 hours.

c) Remove chuck roast from slow cooker, shred with a fork, and return to the slow cooker. Stir meat to evenly coat with sauce. Continue cooking approximately 1 hour.

95. Baked Chicken Breast

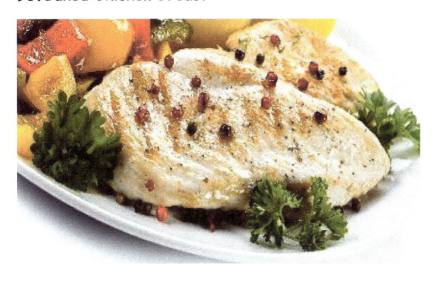

SERVES 10

Ingredients

- 10 boneless skinless chicken breast
- 3/4 cup low-fat yogurt
- 1/2 cup chopped basil
- 2 teaspoons arrowroot flour
- 1 cup oatmeal coarsely ground

Directions

a) Arrange chicken in a baking dish. Combine basil, yogurt and arrowroot flour; mix well and spread over chicken.

b) Mix oatmeal with salt and pepper to taste and sprinkle over chicken.

c) Bake chicken in 375 degrees in the oven for half an hour. Makes 10 servings.

96. Roast Chicken with Rosemary

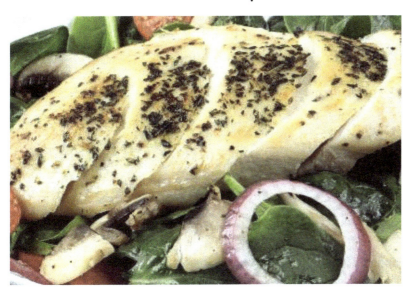

SERVES 6-8

Ingredients

- 1 (3 pound) whole chicken, rinsed, skinned
- salt and pepper to taste
- 1 onion, quartered
- 1/4 cup chopped rosemary

Directions

a) Heat the oven to 350F. Sprinkle salt and pepper on meat. Stuff with the onion and rosemary.

b) Place in a baking dish and bake in the preheated oven until chicken is cooked through.

c) Depending on the size of the bird, cooking time will vary.

97. Carne Asada

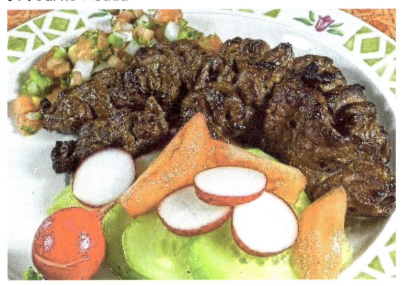

Directions

a) Mix together the garlic, jalapeno, cilantro, salt, and pepper to make a paste. Put the paste in a container. Add the oil, lime juice and orange juice. Shake it up to combine. Use as a marinade for beef or as a table condiment.

b) Put the flank steak in a baking dish and pour the marinade over it. Refrigerate up to 8 hours.
   Take the steak out of the marinade and season it on both sides with salt and pepper.

c) Grill (or broil) the steak for 7 to 10 minutes per side, turning once, until medium-rare. Put the steak on a cutting board and allow the juices to settle (5 minutes). Thinly slice the steak across the grain.

98. Cioppino

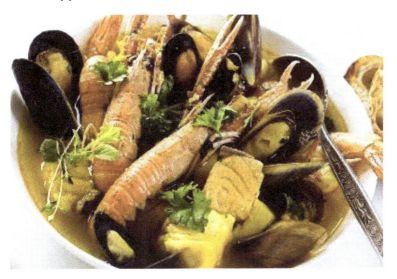

SERVES 6

Ingredients

- 3/4 cup coconut oil
- 2 onions, chopped
- 2 cloves garlic, minced
- 1 bunch fresh parsley, chopped
- 1,5 cups stewed tomatoes
- 1,5 cups chicken broth
- 2 bay leaves
- 1 Tablespoons dried basil
- 1/2 teaspoons dried thyme
- 1/2 teaspoons dried oregano
- 1 cup water
- 1-1/2 cups white wine
- 1-1/2 pounds peeled and deveined large shrimp
- 1-1/2 pounds bay scallops
- 18 small clams
- 18 cleaned and de-bearded mussels
- 1-1/2 cups crabmeat
- 1-1/2 pounds cod fillets, cubed

Directions

a) Over medium heat melt coconut oil in a large stockpot and add onions, parsley and garlic. Cook slowly, stirring occasionally until onions are soft. Add tomatoes to the pot. Add chicken broth, oregano, bay leaves, basil, thyme, water and wine. Mix well.

b) Cover and simmer 30 minutes.
   Stir in the shrimp, scallops, clams, mussels and crabmeat. Stir in fish. Bring to boil. Lower heat, cover and simmer until clams open.

99. Flounder with Orange Coconut

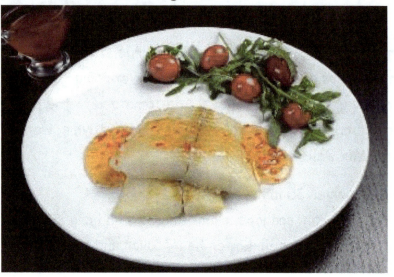

Serves 6

Ingredients

- 3 1/2 lbs. flounder
- 3 Tablespoons white wine
- 3 Tablespoons lemon juice
- 3 Tablespoons coconut oil
- 3 Tablespoons parsley
- 1 teaspoon black pepper
- 2 Tablespoons orange zest
- 1/2 teaspoons salt
- 1/2 cup chopped scallions

Directions

a) Preheat oven to 325F. Sprinkle fish with pepper and salt.

b) Place fish in the baking dish. Sprinkle orange zest on top of the fish. Melt remaining coconut oil and add the parsley and scallions to the coconut oil and pour over flounder. Then add in the white wine.

c) Place in oven and bake for 15 minutes. Serve fish with extra juice on a side.

100. Grilled Salmon

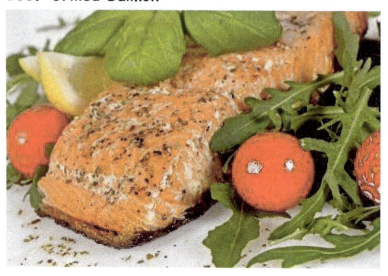

Serves 4

Ingredients

- 4 (4 ounce) filets salmon
- 1/4 cup coconut oil
- 2 Tablespoons fish sauce
- 2 Tablespoons lemon juice
- 2 Tablespoons thinly sliced green onion
- 1 clove garlic, minced and 3/4 teaspoons ground ginger
- 1/2 teaspoons crushed red pepper flakes
- 1/2 teaspoons sesame oil
- 1/8 teaspoons salt

Directions

a) Whisk together coconut oil, fish sauce, garlic, ginger, red chili flakes, lemon juice, green onions, sesame oil, and salt. Put fish in a glass dish, and pour marinade over.

b) Cover and refrigerate for 4 hours.

c) Preheat grill. Place salmon on grill. Grill until fish becomes tender. Turn halfway during cooking.

CONCLUSION

To determine if a food is low fat, a person can read its nutrition label. It is vital to read the part of the label that lists specific values, as many manufacturers label foods as "low fat" despite them having a relatively high fat content.

Examples of low fat foods a person can incorporate into their diet include:

- Cereals, grains, and pasta products
- corn or whole wheat tortillas
- baked crackers
- most cold cereals
- noodles, especially whole grain versions
- oatmeal
- rice
- whole grain bagels
- English muffins
- pita bread